KNEE PAIN:
KNOW MORE

*The key to the knee
is understanding the VMO*

HEDLEY PIPER, FRCS

THE CHOIR PRESS

First published in the United Kingdom in 2023 by
The Choir Press

ISBN 978-1-78963-345-0

Acknowledgements

To the team at The Choir Press I express my gratitude, in particular to David's encouragement and patience. There is a Kevin somewhere in Los Angeles who has shown admirable forbearance as he helped with the initial formatting that took my jumbled notes to a readable format. And friend Donna, who tore it all apart one night, much to the benefit of the reader. I thank you all. And, of course, to Ruth, my wife, who gets her kitchen table back.

Contents

List of Illustrations   vii

Preface   ix

Foreword   xi

Introduction   xiii

Section 1   Background and Problems   1

Chapter 1   Premises   2

Chapter 2   Approach to Knee Pain   3

Chapter 3   Backgrounds and Training   6

Chapter 4   Orthopaedics and Physiotherapy   9

Chapter 5   Pain Inhibition and Coordination: The Basics   13

Section 2   Fast Track   15

Chapter 6   Fast Track: The VMO Exercise   20

Chapter 7   Fast Track: Rehabilitation at Home   35

Section 3   The Science   43

Chapter 8   Application of Basic Science: Anatomy, Physiology
             and Pathology   44

Chapter 9   Anatomy of the Leg Bones and the Angles Involved   51

Chapter 10   Anatomy of the Quadricep Muscles and the Vastus
             Medialis Oblique   57

Chapter 11   Nerve Supply to the Quadriceps   65

Chapter 12   Articular Surfaces   79

Chapter 13   The Patella   87

Chapter 14   How Pain Seems to Work   96

Chapter 15   The Mechanisms of Extension of the Knee   103

Chapter 16   Movements and Functions: Considerations in
             Human Knees   105

Section 4   Common Conditions and Notes on their Management   117

Chapter 17 Origins of Pains from the Knee   118
Chapter 18 The Teenage Knee (and a bit beyond). Conditions
            seen in Teenagers   133
Chapter 19 Adult Anterior Knee Pains   143
Chapter 20 Stability in the Knee Joint   150
Chapter 21 Sport-related Knee Problems   154
Chapter 22 Hamstrings: A Note   160
Chapter 23 Genu Varus and OA Surgical Options: HTO to
            Hemi-arthroplasty   161

**Section 5   Notes for the Health Care Practioner's Attention
               and to Raise the Patient's Expectations as to
               What Might be Reasonably Expected**   177

Appendix: Some Surgical Procedures and Reflections Thereon   187
Glossary of Terms   192
Author Biography   198

List of Illustrations

Fig 1   Bone alignment: the Carrying Angle   16
Fig 2   Quads attachment to femur   17
Fig 3   To illustrate the 'Q' Angle   17
Fig 4   Contrast the 'Q' Angle and the Carrying Angle   18
Fig 5   The Dummy Pass; the 'Q' Angle   19
Fig 6   VMO correction force   21
Fig 7   VMO correction force 4   22
Fig 8   Anatomy of the thigh   23
Fig 9   VMO correction force 2   25
Fig 10   Summary of VMO anatomy and function   26
Fig 11   Position for the isometric VMO exercise   28
Fig 12   Diagram given to patients in clinic after receiving
          VMO instructions   34
Fig 13   Bathroom scales trick: weighing the leg   35
Fig 14   Progressive step-up exercises   36
Fig 15   Elevation of legs   39
Fig 16   The meaning of 'varus' and 'valgus'   52
Fig 17   To illustrate the 'Q' Angle   54
Fig 18   Contrast the 'Q' Angle and the Carrying Angle   55
Fig 19   Quads attachment to femur   53
Fig 20   Anatomy of the thigh   56
Fig 21   VMO anatomy and function as stabiliser of the knee   59
Fig 22   Pressure and shear at the joint line between the patella
          and the femur   60
Fig 23   Anatomy of the femoral nerve   65
Fig 24   The large nerve to the VMO entering the muscle belly   67
Fig 25   Section of nerve bundle to the VMO at the distal thigh,
          low power   68
Fig 26   Nerve bundle to the VMO as it enters muscle; one bundle
          from Fig 25 at high power   69
Fig 27   The leash of nerves forming the femoral nerve in the groin
          without the nerve to the VMO   70
Fig 28   Leash of femoral nerve fibres at the inguinal ligament,
          low power   71

Fig 29   One of the nerves from the leash to the powerhouse muscles
          at the inguinal ligament from Fig 28, high power   72
Fig 30   Anatomy of the femoral nerve   76
Fig 31   How fluid is squeezed out as pressure is applied to hyaline
          cartilage and how it goes back in as pressure is relieved   80
Fig 32   Hyaline cartilage   80
Fig 33   The cartilage matrix   81
Fig 34   Pressure in contact surfaces   89
Fig 35   Skyline diagram of the patellofemoral joint   90
Fig 36   Hunter's cap patellae   91
Fig 37   Position for getting a skyline patellar view X-ray film   92
Fig 38   Bipartate patella   95
Fig 39   Cross section of the spinal chord   101
Fig 40   Rollback   106
Fig 41   Pivot shift   107
Fig 42   The medial wedge for runners   108
Fig 43   Meniscus problems   121
Fig 44   Pivot shift   122
Fig 45   Rollback   140
Fig 46   Runner's medial wedge   155
Fig 47   Single leg squats   156
Fig 48   High valgus tibial osteotomy   162
Fig 49   Hemi marmor prosthesis   165
Fig 50   Patelloplasty   167
Fig 51   Elevation and realignment of the tibial tubercle   168
Fig 52   Pivot shift   181
Fig 53   Langer's lines   191

Preface

The overall aim of a book like this is to inform. The information is useful and not generally well distributed. My audience, I think, should be broad. I do recognise the difficulty to interest both the layman and the professional. The initial drive came from my handling of the anterior knee pains of youth—chondromalacia patellae, as it is called—which I found very easy to treat, and yet others seemed to make its management complicated and expensive. The principles herein can be applied to all knee rehabilitation. The unpublished anatomical studies and their implications, which are included, should be seriously considered by the orthopaedic and physiotherapy worlds. The lay person with 'Knee Pain' can help themselves and can now 'Know More'.

Knee pain is common; detailed knowledge is not. The implications of the very much larger size of the nerve supplying the vastus medialis oblique muscle (VMO) is that this muscle primarily has fine control functions rather than simply power function. It requires a different rehabilitation regimen to power muscles and seems more susceptible to the inhibitory effects of pain.

A word of warning to the lay reader: in academic circles 'anecdote' has become almost a dirty word. Nothing can even be considered if it has not passed the test of the double blind-clinical trial. And yet the 'scientific method' is based on observation. If most cases do well and a couple do not, the intelligent practitioner stops and asks: 'What factors did I not consider that changed the outcome?' Over 35 years as a surgeon, I have observed the orthopaedic world struggle with the management of knee problems.

My prime aim is to try to improve the advice given for the rehabilitation of knees. My secondary aim is to give people on both ends of the knife more understanding of what could be wrong—in medical parlance, the 'differential diagnosis'—and to form strategies to help in the diagnosis, treatment and recovery. By learning to better use their vastus medialis oblique muscle, people should be able to gain some relief from their sore knees and more rapid recovery after surgical intervention. There is instruction and there is science to back this up. And there are things that one could expect from one's treating professional.

Disclaimer: The reader must accept responsibility for their medical care and treatment. The author cannot be held responsible for failure to fully understand the insights offered in this book. In no circumstances can the publisher or the author accept any legal responsibility or liability for any loss or damage arising from any error in or omission from the information contained in this book, or from the failure of the reader to properly follow any instruction contained in the book.

Foreword

As a surgeon, I include a few surgical pearls and some fairly strong opinions based on many years of reading and surgical practice. Some I have tried to confine to the 'small print', or to the later sections directed more towards the professional. As a consultant specialist in a wide general orthopaedic practice, my role was not simply to make the diagnosis—which is usually not very demanding—nor simply to be the technician and do the operation, but to try to eliminate, as far as possible, all other possibilities, which meant that not infrequently I would test hoping for negative findings as much as for positive findings (in backs, for example). Sadly, the iatrogenic effects of testing can be profoundly negative. 'Iatrogenic' means caused by the medical processes or environment (from the Greek 'iatros', meaning doctor). Testing causes anxiety and confusion because of false positives and, occasionally, false negatives. But in our medico-legal-aware world, failure to test can be expensive. The practitioner must overprotect himself and his institution by over testing and worrying a lot of families, and potentially costing a lot of money.

If a knee has pain, a consistent storyline or history—for example, it locks or blocks from time to time, gives way unexpectedly, has turned into a 'rice crispy', meaning that it has developed a 'snap', a 'crackle' or a 'pop', and, most importantly, on clinical examination it has an effusion (fluid in the joint)—this means that somewhere inside, that knee is not happy. And this really is the indication for an arthroscopy, without further expensive investigations!

There are routine tests that are a necessary part of any initial consultation. Simple radiographs (X-rays to the layman and me) with one or two special views—an AP Weight-bearing view, always; sometimes a Skyline Patellar view; even on occasion a Through the Notch view— plus a good clinical examination is really all that is needed to make an educated diagnosis. No amount of testing or scanning thereafter can do anything to help cure the problem. The findings on arthroscopy are not always consistent with the scan, CT or MRI. Presupposing that the arthroscopist is competent, one can with an arthroscope not only confirm the diagnosis but immediately carry on to treat the problems, or at the very least plan a sensible strategy of management.

There are really two groups of patients: those who do not need a surgeon—their problem will settle with rehabilitation and possible medication—and those with a pathology that only a doctor or surgeon can address. However, both groups will benefit from intelligent rehabilitation. Many knee pains, particularly in the younger age groups, do not need a surgical procedure. They really do not need investigation, nor any special braces or orthotics, but they do need the rehabilitation ideas set out in this book, which will cure them. Not a few elderly folk have declared that getting their VMO working again has helped them greatly.

(NB I have tried to write with normal print for the storyline, italics for detailed techniques that the professional might find useful, and footnotes and small print for details that the lay reader may wish to skip, or that they might use to challenge their carer.)

The first section is the background and logic underpinning some of my recommendations. The second section, 'Fast Track', is what you would get in my clinic: some understanding. The third section is the turgid science. The fourth section is what you should expect from your carer. The fifth section are notes on common conditions and knee problems. The Appendix contains some interventions for the surgeon to ponder. Within each section are the numbered chapter headings for clarity.

I have included unpublished observations on the anatomy of the nerve to the vastus medialis oblique and the important implications they have on the understanding and the rehabilitation of knees.

The information is accurate.[1] Some of it is opinionated. There may be disagreement from many practitioners; however, the science behind my views has been borne out and is out there and published in the public domain for the diligent reader, should they so choose. The exceptions are the microscopic cross-sections of the nerve to the vastus medialis oblique and the inferences to be made from them.

---

[1] While this is a serious tome based on science, I deliberately have not tried to compile a long list of references. There is a vast body of writings out there, some more sensible than others. I do not expect the lay reader to bother to read them. The diligent professional should already have read most of them as part of their training.

Introduction

There are many books and many pundits, but not so many experts. This is true in many fields; the knee is no exception.

Despite all that is preached and written, knees continue to give great pain and discomfort and limit the mobility of a lot of people, generating a great deal of work for health professionals: surgeons, physiotherapists, sports medicine hacks, and even the odd 'Uncle Tom Cobley'. There are huge vested interests in the medical management of knee problems, so reader beware, and be careful unto whom you listen.

To this end, I wish to make a small offering that does not echo the crowds but looks at the problems of knee pains and their rehabilitation with a rather different approach that may challenge some of the commonly held ideas.

I have written bits of this over many years of orthopaedic surgical practice—a chapter here and a thought there, and which repetitions I have tried to eliminate. Sometimes things need repeating; in clinic it was important to repeat the message three times if one wanted the patient to really grasp the idea, and even then I could hear the nurse re-explaining things after I had left the room. *(Oh, and patients cannot hear if they are not wearing their glasses!)*

My recent research into the state of play in knee treatment has surprised me in that some of the ideas in this book are still not yet 'out there'. I am sad to say that there is quite a bit of rubbish being taught: to patients, to physiotherapists, to medical students and to trainee orthopaedic surgeons. One is the idea that one cannot isolate the vastus medialis oblique to train it. Yes, you can. There is a little science that has been underappreciated and therefore not integrated into knee rehabilitation. Well, here it is!

The conscientious knee patient may well have been instructed in a variety of exercises in all sorts of odd postures and which may require more or less apparatus to perform, depending upon the school of treatment to which their therapist adheres. Diligent repetition of some of these exercises may well have helped, although evidently not for many of those patients who presented to me.

The aim is to provide a simple-to-use guide to knee problems and rehabilitation and to offer some understanding of the possible causes for pain and possibilities for relieving it. That the more assertive patients will also have some technical knowledge with which to question their carers may, or may not, be a benefit.

I believe that if treatment is simple and gets quick results, it should have good compliance. ('Compliance' is the jargon medical word meaning that the patients do what they have been told to do!) From my experience, with the ideas in this book, people complied and got better. Of course, if it reduces the need for physiotherapy sessions, it may not be popular with all patients, some of whom enjoy the attention. Nor may it be so popular with those health professionals whose income depends on numbers seen. But for those with the knee pain, any small contribution can help.

Yes, I was a surgeon, and yes, there is a very definite place for surgery, particularly in dealing with the root causes for some pains, but there are many situations where simple re-education of the muscles of control of the knee, without any other therapeutic measure, will relieve the problem. If a medical intervention is needed, there still remains the requirement of good rehabilitation of the muscles after the surgical procedure, and that, dear reader, is what this book is about.

To quote Sinclair Lewis: 'Talking shop is the purest and most rapturous form of conversation, and nothing is more agonising than to come across, at a dinner party perhaps, someone with whom one longs to talk shop and have to hold back for social constraints of boring other diners.'

The science part of this book is unashamedly 'shop talk', aimed more at the medical professional, but remember, it is about you—or rather your knee! There is a morbid interest for many in 'knowing', so I make no apologies for including it all. I have taken the precaution to group the chapters: key messages for the self-help brigade, and such science that I think helps in understanding the surgical bits, which is probably only of interest to the professional, although the lay reader might like to tease their surgeon if he is not doing it very well.

(Be not afraid, dear reader, to be a little bit assertive. Surgeons do not always appreciate the challenge ... but they do sometimes need it.)

SECTION 1

Background and Problems

The background and problems of treating knee pain and the
misunderstandings that have led to my recommendations.

———◆———

These ideas for rehabilitation have evolved over the years. As a student and junior doctor, I was on the receiving end of knee surgery twice for torn menisci, or 'cartilages', when my knees would lock. In those days it was open surgery, and in my case on the inner sides of each knee. I can promise you that it was jolly uncomfortable. It was also interesting to me, as a student of these things, that the rate of wasting in my quadricep muscles was very fast—48 hours and my thigh's muscles had shrunk by an inch. I have subsequently confirmed this rapid wasting even in the athlete, and how quickly it recovers when the pain is gone.

I was also fortunate that an elderly rheumatologist put his nose into my hospital room (circa 1971) and showed me the VMO exercise and the use of my finger as 'biofeedback', not that he called it that by name. I regret that I do not recall his name, for in many ways that was the key to my thinking over the years.

I used these principles to treat patients in the Western Canadian bush from 1974 to 1978, where there was virtually no out-patient physiotherapy; the distances were just too great. They all had to exercise at home. I have used the same exercises on myself, my family and my patients, who all seemed to get better quite quickly. My wife even heard them being explained and demontrated by a girl to her friends while teaching at a college in Montreal, attributed, I am pleased to say, to one Dr Piper. Teenage anterior knee pains never seemed to me to be a problem, which was not quite the view of many orthopaedic surgeons and physiotherapists.

I am therefore guilty of reasoning back from empirical observation of making patients better via the known sciences to the opinions that I express: for example, the healing of articular cartilage or the existence of the Vastus Medialis Oblique muscle as an entity. There are also some gross over-simplifications in the book, such as how pain seems to work, of which I am well aware.

Chapter 1

Premises

There are a couple of themes that underpin this book:

- **Pain inhibits muscle coordination.**
- **A lot of pain can be experienced from a very small bit of tissue.**
- **Do not confuse muscle re-education with muscle strengthening.**

And an observation:

- **Get the muscle control right, and many of the perceived problems and pains just seem to settle down, without any other measures.**

With knee pain, must one rush to seek medical opinion? Well, no. Unfortunately, you may not be getting sound advice. There most definitely is a place for diagnosis by a 'pro'. The identification of the precise source of the pain is necessary in many knees. Analgaesics (painkillers), non-steroidal anti-inflammatory medications (NSAIDs—'D' because Americans say 'drugs') and injected anti-inflammatory steroids all have their place. Surgery in one form or other may be the only real management solution; it is the role of the clinician to decide. But with or without a surgical intervention, one still needs correct rehabilitation focused on the muscles that control the joint. And for many patients that alone is sufficient to relieve them of their problem.

Chapter 2

Approach to Knee Pain

Diagnosing and treating knee pain has been a problem of management for many; I think because rehabilitation has been a bit hit and miss. Here I am trying to bring together a lot of ideas: the sciences of understanding pain and its inhibitory effects on motor coordination; the anatomy of the quadricep muscles and their nervous innervation, and in particular the vastus medialis oblique; the anatomy of the leg bones; the mechanics of the knee movements and the forces generated by the muscle groups; the science of hyaline cartilage nourishment and damage and the possible things that can go wrong; and even what the medical world should be doing about it. It sounds a lot! Lay reader, please don't panic. I have tried to lay it out in sections into which you can dig as deep as you wish. There are lots of diagrams to help with the explanations.

Section 1   The background.

Section 2   The 'fast track' for those who just want to crack on. It is what you would get in my clinic, enough knowledge to be able to understand what you are trying to do, and then how to do it.

Section 3   The science underlying my suggestions and recommendations in reasonable detail, to which I ask the reader to refer if they do not fully understand.

Section 4   These are what the doctor and physiotherapist can do, or can be expected to do.

Section 5   Different diagnoses for the lay reader to understand and to silence the critics.

Appendix   Procedures for the professional to ponder.

As a patient, one may have pain in a knee—intermittent, stabbing or chronic grumbling— generalised or localised to one spot that you may not think of as anterior. And I agree; a painful knee can just be jolly painful. However, the ideas in this book are all germane to the process of rehabilitation before and after your physician or surgeon has removed or mitigated your agony.

I have tried to offer direction to the processes of diagnosis. As a surgeon, I could stick in needles and inject or aspirate, prescribe medications or arthroscope, order tests, simple or sophisticated, and operate and replace as the need arose. But in each case the rehabilitation in my hands focused on the rehabilitation of the vastus medialis oblique, the steering muscle, rather than the powerhouse muscles or the hamstrings. Get the VMO working correctly and the rest seem to fall into line.

Synergy: the summation of therapies

After one presentation one of my juniors made the point that the message he had picked up was the concept of combining therapies for the summation of effect. I remember that it was not quite what I had meant to get over to them, but he was right.

> Synergy is where things help each other, and summation of effect is when they add up, one plus one making a lot more than two. Example: the man whose wife sends him down 'to clear out the garage'. Small chance. He will get distracted by something. She cannot do it by herself; things are just too heavy. But woe betide the poor chap if his wife comes down with him; the job is done by coffee break!

The same is true for knees. The physician's role is to identify and eliminate as far as possible the root causes of the pain messages. (Perhaps I should point out that the sources of pain in the knee, particularly in the adolescent knee, are not entirely obvious. I discuss them below.) This may require correction of any mechanical problems, and this usually means surgery, plus chemical control of the inflammatory response and analgesia for pain relief with medications. In my practice they were oral medications[2]: analgesia, non-steroidal anti-inflammatory medication, special medication for a disease such as rheumatoid arthritis or gout plus a possible initial intra-articular injection of an anti-inflammatory steroid to start things improving.

Today there are people injecting various things, like hyaluronic acid. I have no experience of them. (Hyaluronic acid, by the way, is a molecule that is important to the lubrication of joints and is integral to the structure of the hyaline cartilage surfaces.)

---

[2] In France suppositories were more popular; in Canada their prescription could empty the clinic!

Re-education of the muscles is always possible but is much more effective when all pathologies[3] are addressed. There are iatrogenic[4] effects to be aware of: some patients like the attention or getting out of classes; various pills may have been prescribed; and there is a lucrative industry in investigations and in supplying braces of various descriptions.

Hospitals tend to produce instruction leaflets—not always very accurate—telling patients what to do and how and when to take their pain medications. Patient, beware! If you do not need painkillers, as directed by the paperwork or the doctor, do not take them. If the hot redness of your sore inflamed knee has settled down, reduce or stop taking the NSAIDs if they are upsetting your stomach; although, if you are suppressing a synovial disease like rheumatoid arthritis or gout, you will need to stay on those medications until your rheumatologist tells you to reduce or stop. But the one thing you do not stop doing is practising the action of your VMO muscle!

This advice—the other way round for the treating physician—in the situation of an intra-articular injection of steroid, for example, is also to give an NSAID for a few days, plus the referral to physiotherapy (i.e. add the modalities). And physiotherapists, please do not stop the medications 'to see if your treatment is working', as has occurred to my patients in the past. The patients get very confused. Recall, please, that the patient sees the surgeon for five minutes once or twice and the physiotherapist for 40 minutes three times a week. And while it may seem brutal, or politically insensitive. to say it, traditional physiotherapy teaching has, like traditional orthopaedics, failed to understand that which is laid out in this book. Please; we all need to be on the same page or it becomes very confusing for patients.

---

[3] 'Pathology' is the medical term for something being wrong with a tissue, or tissues, of the body.
[4] 'Iatrogenic', I have already told you: the medical environment effect. *Iatros* means a doctor in Greek.

Chapter 3

Backgrounds and Training

'Experience is gained through making errors. Making errors is due to
lack of experience.'
(I am sure that a lot of people over the ages have said something similar.
I would not dream of attributing it.)

'Art in medicine is the perception and manipulation of parameters
that science cannot measure.'
(That I attribute to myself!)

One must clinically examine one's patients and not just jump to testing.

Mine was the generation of surgeons who first had to become physicians.
We then had to learn the fine detail of the basic sciences—anatomy,
physiology and pathology—while getting exposure to multiple surgical
disciplines. Only then, after something of a stress test—those long hours as
junior doctors actually examining sick patients—did we specialise in our
chosen branches of surgery. After that we were told: 'Go forth and put it all
into practice.' And we did. We experimented.

Our experimental animal walked on two legs. I can recall being a bit
uneasy about that. Up to the end of the 1960s there were publications of
new ideas. Then the risks of being associated with an idea that did not pan
out became too great for the academics, and medical and surgical
publications become more cautious and increasingly just series of results
with tentative discussion and conclusions.

It is not quite the same today. There are masses of publications out there.
Some of the wide general experience of training seems to have been
dropped. Being a holistic physician seems not to be so important; 'Make
the diagnosis, classify it, learn the cookbook, apply the recipe' seems to be
the thrust of so much of today's training. It is worth noting that my
generation had about 30,000 hours of surgical experience in the operating
room, and the concomitant hours in clinics and on the wards, before being
appointed consultant. Those who could not take the stress of the long hours
dropped out. Today's surgical trainee in the UK is lucky to have 6,000 hours
of surgery prior to appointment as a surgeon; better supervised perhaps, but
much less clinic and ward experience.

I also benefitted from a period as a resident at McGill University in Montreal. The focus on reading and theoretical knowledge was intense, but because the North American systems pay the surgeon per item of work, the opportunities for residents to actually get to operate alone was much more limited. In the 1960s and 1970s Antipodeans—Australians, New Zealanders and not a few South Africans—would come to Britain as part of their training because they could 'cut'. I met some who after a year or two in a slow practice back home would come back to the UK and take a locum position for a few months to regain their confidence and 'cut a few more Poms'![5]

Manual skills require practice. I always felt that in choosing one's dentist one should look in his garage; in his chair your head is back, your mouth is open and you cannot talk nor see what he is doing. He could be doing anything! Anaesthesia used to take a few minutes. Now it seems to take up hours, anaesthetists please note. The throughput varies greatly as a result, with late starts and early finishes, holiday leave and study leave, which all reduces the amount of practise of manual surgical dexterity an individual surgeon can get.

The new health-care management[6] view is that you, the public, are no longer simply patients; you are clients and customers, and your enjoyment of the experience is about all that is measured. There seems to be very little measurement of outcomes, or skills and effectiveness of individual surgeons, nor even the generation of costs by different practices. It is very difficult to know just how good, technically, somebody really is. A well-informed patient can at least challenge sensibly the advice of their carer. This book is to try to promote some understanding of the management of knee pain, on both sides!

Choosing a surgeon is difficult

At a cocktail party he will always be the 'best man', 'the top man in his field'. There is probably a big vested interest in having paid the chap. In choosing one's surgeon, his technical skill is really all you should be interested in, not his bedside manner, not his reputation from all the academic papers he has published, nor the committees he has chaired. In doing all that, he would not have had the time to practise his manual dexterity! You want the surgeon whose only interest is his own batting average. That is the man who is going to do the best job. Your knee is, after all, just another bit of grist in his mill.

---

[5] 'Poms' is a mildly derogatory Australian term for the British, something to do with using pomegranate as an anti scorbutic.
[6] 'Management' is what we medics call the overall treatment of a patient; not to be confused with the hospital administration.

How do you find out this sort of information. It is very difficult, even for myself, unless you happen to know the theatre staff, who can tell you who is technically capable or who they would want as their surgeon. As a lay person you have to be just a bit more assertive and ask the surgeon, 'As a good technician, which procedure do you use?' or 'Which incision ...?'

Chapter 4

Orthopaedics and Physiotherapy

'Orthopaedic' means 'straight child' in Greek. Today it is about aches and pains and physical injury. Physiotherapy, physically moving and training bits of people's bodies, started between the 1914/18 and 1939/45 wars, helping wounded soldiers to recover.

Osteomyelitis is a staphylococcus infection in bones, often in children; tuberculosis is another bacterial infection that attacked joints. Until after the Second World War there were no antibiotics. TB and osteomyelitis were relatively common problems years ago. They are painful conditions. The management of such infections was surgical: the opening and drainage of the sites and months and years of convalescence, which is why many orthopaedic hospitals were sited outside of the town centres in what was then still countryside, as clean air and good food were about the only thing that could be offered.

Infections can be very painful. Chronic pain causes people, particularly children, to curl up and their muscles to go into spasm and eventually shorten. This produced sore, stiff, curled-up children with fixed flexion deformities. The same thing occurred in adults, but without the complication of growth.

When straightening these children with orthopaedic procedures, surgeons used surgical drainage and surgical releases, where one has to cut muscle ligaments and tendons. This was followed by bedrest with splints and traction for months and even years, while the body healed the infection by what is called 'secondary intention'.[7]

Physical therapy was needed to keep muscles and joints working and to regain their range of motion during and after the infection was controlled. Re-education of the movements was needed as patients got up and tried to get about. And, thus, physiotherapy and rehabilitation became a speciality.

During the Second World War and immediately afterwards there was an epidemic of poliomyelitis. This disease was endemic in the Middle East and has a predilection for young adults. It was the troops who brought it back from that area. The end result of polio is that motor nerve cells in the spinal cord are destroyed. Muscles without their motor nerves are paralysed. The

---

[7] Secondary intention is the slow process of healthy tissues gradually growing over and filling up the wound.

paralysis is permanent. The orthopaedic hospitals were the places of choice for these patients, as they were geared up for the care of long-term, bed-bound patients. Physiotherapy was essential to their rehabilitation and recovery.

Derivative information can be dangerous

Derivative information is something that has been published and subsequently copied from textbook to textbook without being challenged and verified. It has become an 'alternative truth'. It may well have been wrong. Knee rehabilitation has suffered from this. I shall explain.

The rationale behind the methods of rehabilitation

Surgeons treating injured and paralysed patients developed operations to stabilise joints, drain abscesses, transfer tendons to overcome paralysed functions and generally try to get people going again. The understanding of the management of the paralysis of poliomyelitis, spinal injury, spina bifida and fixed deformities was important, for the same principles can also be applied to trauma and reconstruction.

It was realised very quickly that tendon transfers had to be in the same phase for the patient to be able to learn to use it (i.e. for a flexor function one must use a flexor tendon and/or muscle, and for extensor function one must find an extensor tendon and/or muscle). Otherwise, the patients found it almost impossible to use the 'restored' function.

Dr Jacqueline Perry, MD, worked in the Ranchos Los Amigos Rehabilitation Center, California, in the late 1940s, the 1950s and the 1960s and wrote extensively on rehabilitation, including the knee. Much of her work is the basis of many physiotherapy textbooks. But alas, she got this one vital thing very wrong. When re-educating the use of muscles, they must all be worked in the same phase. Her recommendations for knee rehabilitation ignored this phase requirement and are an example of derivative information that is not correct but gets copied from textbook to textbook without challenge. I wish to attempt to correct that error.

It is important to emphasise here the difference: that instruction for muscle re-education or training must be in the same phase. Instruction for increasing muscle power seems less sensitive and is more related to ADLs (activities of daily living) where there is the normal coordination of extensor and flexor functions.

This basic principle of remaining in the same phase—using a flexor for flexor function and an extensor to restore extensor function—is very necessary for a patient to relearn to use muscles. Some of Dr Perry's recommendations for knee rehabilitation, in particular lifting the straight leg at the hip and pulling the foot up at the ankle—both of which are flexor phase—while extending the knee with quadricep contraction—which is extensor function—mix the two phases. This mixture of demands of flexor and extensor function at the same time occurs in normal movements, but it is not helpful when relearning a specific fine control function. It is why a lot of knee exercises take a long time to achieve improvement or just do not work.

Patterning

Physiotherapy and neurological textbooks used to make much of this, particularly in the assessment of head-injury patients. There is a whole plethora of muscle-control reflexes that are spinal, which is how we can wander around not paying too much attention—running up and down stairs and generally doing 'stuff'—and we do not keep falling over. If we become decerebrate (i.e. our hind brain and spinal cord are not functionally connected to our cerebral cortex, as after a severe head injury), when there are no motor messages being sent to the spinal cord, the body assumes a position with the arms in unopposed flexion and the legs in pure extension. This is called 'patterning'. It is well recognised. The extended leg has the foot pointing down and inverted.

Doing exercises for muscle training in the correct phase position very much relates to patterning. ADLs are driven by motor impulses sent down the spinal cord from our cerebral cortex that act upon the spinal reflexes. Brain thinks, 'Put my hand out, point my finger and touch ...' and sends out some signals, but it does not have to worry about overbalancing or continuing to stand upright, push with triceps and let out biceps or even that the shoulder might be moving with every breath. This is all taken care of by the spinal reflexes. Trying to integrate an out-of-phase muscle into a hard-wired pattern of movement, patients found very difficult. Patterning dictates the required position for performing quadricep re-educating exercises: pure extension of the leg; remember that tibialis posterior is a powerful extensor and inverter of the foot. We shall come to this.

Perhaps I should apologise to physiotherapists. They are a very necessary part of the team, but this failure of their textbooks to emphasise phase in rehabilitation is an important lacuna, particularly in relation to the knee.

The other message of this book, the failure to appreciate the implications of the size and components of the nerve to vastus medialis oblique, is hardly a fault confined to physiotherapists. Orthopaedic surgeons are just as guilty. I shall explain in detail elsewhere.

I have stated that the great premise of this book is that pain alters coordination. Running a close second is the idea that one does not need a big bit of damaged tissue to have a lot of pain. They bear repeating.

Try sticking a sewing needle into one's knee and see what it feels like. It is worse than a jab in the finger. (Actually, it is easier to use someone else's knee.) It is a very small injury and would be invisible on the inside if one has an arthroscope in the joint. But the effect would be very painful, and they, or you, would limp. A limp is a failure to coordinate muscles normally. Yet the needle got nowhere near the muscles. It is the pain messages feeding back and altering the normal spinal reflex controls of movement that cause the limp.

The thing for we physicians and surgeons is to consider what could be the source of a patient's pain and to understand its effects, and to know what to do to remove that source and how to mitigate the effects of the pain. Seems simple, so why the problems? Read on.

Chapter 5

Pain Inhibition and Coordination: The Basics

I have just stated that this book is based on a couple of important ideas:

a) Pain inhibits good muscle coordination.
b) One does not need a big bit of tissue damage to get a lot of pain, and therefore a lot of inhibitory feedback.

These are key to understanding the problems of the knee. A pinprick into a knee can cause limping.

What is limping? It is simply poor coordination of the muscles of locomotion, induced in this case by a painful pin prick. The tissues that would be damaged would be the skin, the fibrous capsule of the joint and the synovium, but not the muscles. Synovium is particularly sensitive to pain. It is the pain that inhibits the reflex control of the muscles. One can consciously override a limp. But consider just how much or little tissue was actually damaged by the pin—very little, and yet a very big effect. If one puts a needle into a joint during an arthroscopy and then removes it and looks for the entry wound on the inside, it is impossible to see the hole—and arthroscopes magnify.

So in certain circumstances we need not postulate that it takes a big bit of injured or sensitive tissue to have a painful experience. One cannot necessarily see the actual site that may be the source of pain. In the case of anterior knee pain in adolescent girls investigated with arthroscopy in the 1970s, people could find no source of damage, although there were occasionally reports of a little pinkness of the synovium on the medial side of the patella; but then most people used exsanguination (squeezing the blood out) of the leg and applied a tourniquet, so any increased blood flow in an inflamed synovium would not be very apparent.

(I do sometimes wonder whether if someone had jabbed a needle into the knee of the surgeon declaring that he could 'see nothing untoward' in the adolescent's knee, thinking might have been different—that a very small injury can cause a lot of discomfort.)

Every athlete knows that a little pain interferes with good coordination; most call it 'stiffness'. An ambitious 17-year-old second row forward (rugby!) was asked how he would handle a particularly capable opposite number. After due consideration, his reply was, ''Urt 'im!' He was indeed a very perceptive young man.

In the knee, the muscle most susceptible to the inhibitory effect of pain is the steering muscle, that fine control muscle, the vastus medialis oblique. It is the inability of this muscle to overcome the lateral shear force on the patella, generated for the most part by the main powerhouse muscles of the quadriceps—the vastus lateralis, the vastus intermedius and the vastus medialis (not the vastus medialis oblique)—which causes the conditions that lead to anterior knee pain, certainly in youth, and contributes to knee pain in adults.

Quadricep Incoordination Syndrome (QIS)

Incoordination of the quadriceps, secondary to pain inhibition, is the common thread in knee problems and rehabilitation. QIS (Quadricep Incoordination Syndrome) should really have been described. It really exists. In the 1970s and 1980s everyone was describing a new syndrome. QIS is simply poor coordination of the steering muscle—the vastus medialis oblique—with the powerhouse bulk of the quadriceps, and is sufficient to cause knee pain. This incoordination is a surprisingly common finding on careful clinical examination of adults by just asking the patient to contract their thigh muscles; the VMO lags behind the power quads. It is also simple to treat by re-education of VMO function.

Any condition that is painful will have an incoordination-producing effect. If, when attempting to treat knee pain, one can identify a specific site of pain or a mechanical cause of discomfort, it must be addressed or it will constantly be working against attempts at rehabilitation. Very often the patient is in a vicious-circle situation: pain causing inhibition and incoordination, which is causing the pain. This is particularly true in the adolescent.

SECTION 2

Fast Track

'The stronger the body, the more it obeys; the weaker the body,
the more it commands.'

Jean-Jacques Rousseau
1712–1778

———•———

This is the basic information and instruction that I would give you in clinic to start the rehabilitation of your knee and thigh muscles. It is aimed at the 'self-help' brigade.

The Carrying Angle is the fixed angle made by the line of the femoral shaft and the tibial shaft. It is greater in women than in men. The thigh muscles pulling on the kneecap arise from these bones.

In young children there is little difference between the angles in boys and girls. However, as the pelvis widens in girls at puberty, the hips are carried outwards, but the knees stay together, so the angle must increase. The femoral heads are also smaller and the femoral neck is shorter. The angle becomes fixed as the growth epiphyses fuse. It is the changing coordination required of the quadriceps during the growth spurt that is the trigger for adolescent knee pain.

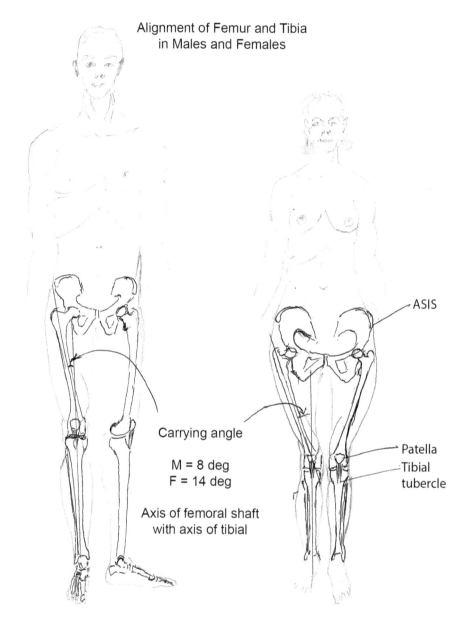

Alignment of Femur and Tibia
in Males and Females

ASIS

Carrying angle

M = 8 deg
F = 14 deg

Axis of femoral shaft
with axis of tibial

Patella
Tibial
tubercle

N.B. The 'Q' Angle is dynamic. It is the line from the ASIS to the patella and the patella to the tibial tubercle. There is rotation at the knee which changes the 'Q' Angle.

Fig 1 Bone alignment: the Carrying Angle

The alignment of the quadriceps, patella and patellar tendon is very dynamic during movement. The angle in the pulley system changes constantly with the degree of rotation of the tibia under the femoral condyles. Often it is called the 'Q' Angle, which, misleadingly for some, seems to imply that it is something rather fixed; in fact, it is constantly changing. The angles in the pulley system are higher in women than in men because of the shapes of their bones.

The Carrying Angle is the fixed angle in each individual's legs between the line of the femur (thigh) and the line of the tibia (shin).

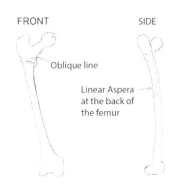

Fig 2 Quads attachment to femur

The muscle attachments of the power-producing quadriceps are all lateral to the patella; they are on the anterior, lateral and posterior aspects of the proximal third of the femur.

The 'Q' Angle is constantly changing because during movement there is not only bending and straightening at the knee; there is also rotation between the tibia and the femur. As we twist and turn, our femur rotates on the tibia. The movements of the subtalar joint in the foot and ankle cause rotation of the tibia under the femoral condyles—germane in the long-distance athlete's knee—and there is also rotation of the femur at the hip as it swings backwards and forwards under the pelvis. All are integral to all movement, even in a straight line. Rotation is more apparent when turning off a planted foot (see Fig 5, page 19).

The angle of the line of pull of the powerhouse element of the quads on the patella, and the patellar tendon attached to the tibia, is always changing slightly, so the effort of the steering muscle must constantly change. (The body weight, alas, may not be so dynamic.)

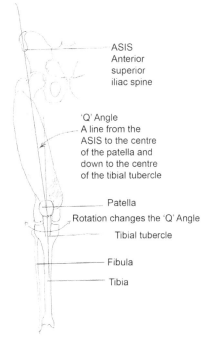

Fig 3 To illustrate the 'Q' Angle

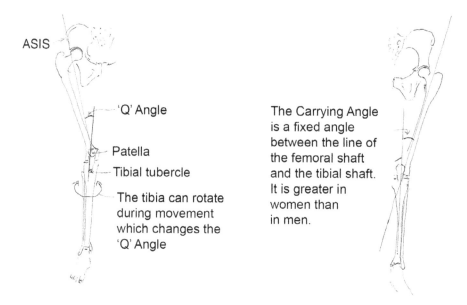

ASIS

'Q' Angle

Patella

Tibial tubercle

The tibia can rotate
during movement
which changes the
'Q' Angle

The Carrying Angle
is a fixed angle
between the line of
the femoral shaft
and the tibial shaft.
It is greater in
women than
in men.

Fig 4 Contrast the 'Q' Angle and the Carrying Angle

Care of the articular surfaces

All moving surfaces of joints are covered in hyaline cartilage, or articular cartilage, terms for the same thing (not to be confused with 'cartilage', as in 'I had my cartilage removed from my knee', when you meant 'meniscus'). Hyaline cartilage needs to be looked after.

Hyaline cartilage works within certain physical limitations. It evolved to work in a limited pressure range and it is directional stuff. (This, by the way, is true in adult hyaline cartilage across the spectrum of all animals.) While cartilage can withstand loads in the direction for which it was evolved, it cannot withstand shear (i.e. sideways) movement, particularly when it is under load. Shear under load causes splitting in the depth of the matrix of the hyaline cartilage and the releasing of PG (proteoglycans) and GAG (glycosaminoglycans).[8] PGs and GAGs stimulate the synovium to overwork, in effect inflammation, which is a cause for pain. The undersurfaces of the patella and the bearing surfaces of the condyles of the femur must survive within these physical tolerances. It is the VMO (vastus medialis oblique) that is supposed to constantly make the multiple, corrective efforts to ensure that the load is always correctly applied.

---

[8] See section on hyaline cartilage, proteoglycans and glycosaminoglycans, Chapter 12.

'Wobble' of the quadricep mass from side to side would compound the pressure problem. I believe that the role of the fascia lata and probably sartorius are primarily to stabilise the quads and prevent wobble and changing load pressures.

A 'clinical' examination, by the way, implies that you, the patient or at least your problem part is formally examined by the clinician. Too often the examination is rather cursory and there is a rush to ordering tests. One could ask after the examination: 'What do you think, Doctor?' before he starts ordering stuff. You can get an idea about their skills by how thorough the clinical examination is.

Definition of 'Q' Angle:
The angle subtended by lines drawn from the anterior superior iliac spine to the centre of the patella and then from the centre of the patella to the middle of the tibial tubercle.

Problem:
There is rotation of the tibia under the femur with almost all movement; every time we twist and turn and also walking on uneven ground and using our subtalar joints to align the feet, all cause some degree of rotation at the knee.

The Dummy Pass

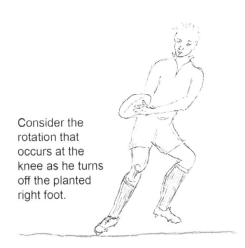

Consider the rotation that occurs at the knee as he turns off the planted right foot.

Fig 5 The Dummy Pass: the 'Q' Angle

Chapter 6

Fast Track: The VMO Exercise

For those who are reading this and wish to crack on, there is just a little understanding to be expected of you. It is easier if you understand what it is you are trying to do.

Look at the diagrams: Fig 1 (page 16), Fig 2 (page 17), Figs 3 and 4 (pages 17 and 18), Fig 5 (page 19). The bones of the legs are angled down from the hips, which are apart, to the knees, which are together. The shin bones then go more or less straight down to the ankles, which are also together. The angle at the knee between the shafts of the thigh bone (femur) and the shin bone (tibia) is greater in women because their hips are further apart. It is called the Carrying Angle, and it does not change.

By contrast, the muscles and tendons, with the patella in the middle, form a pulley system that straightens the knee and is angled: the 'Q' Angle (see Fig 3, page 17).

The 'Q' Angle is defined as from the ASIS (anterior superior iliac spine) to the centre of the patella and then to the tibial tubercle. This angle is very dynamic, changing with almost every movement of walking and running around. It is the vastus medialis oblique's function to produce a medialising force to counterbalance the lateralising force generated by the main power production of the quadricep muscles.

Line of pull of the
powerhouse
muscles

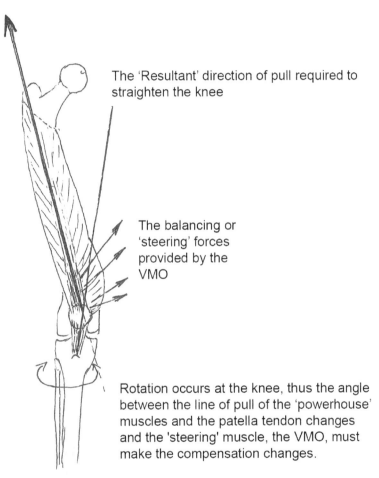

The 'Resultant' direction of pull required to
straighten the knee

The balancing or
'steering' forces
provided by the
VMO

Rotation occurs at the knee, thus the angle
between the line of pull of the 'powerhouse'
muscles and the patella tendon changes
and the 'steering' muscle, the VMO, must
make the compensation changes.

Fig 6 VMO correction force

To show how the VMO corrects the 'bow string' effect of the powerhouse muscles on the patella.

Ideal line of pull on
Patello Femoral Joint

Actual line of pull
of 'powerhouse'

Corrective force of
VMO contraction

Bow string effect

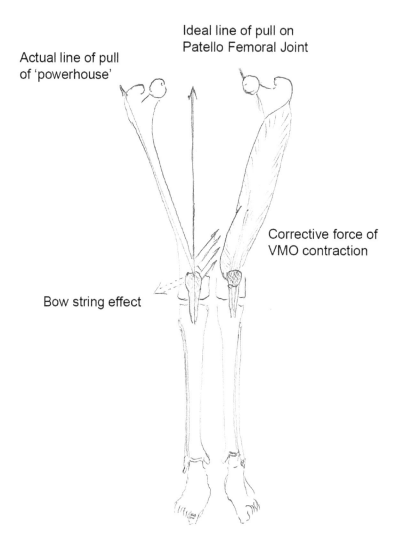

Fig 7 VMO correction force 4

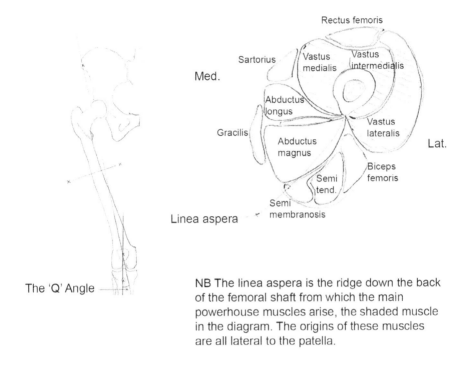

Rectus femoris

Med.

Sartorius

Vastus medialis

Vastus intermedialis

Abductus longus

Gracilis

Abductus magnus

Vastus lateralis

Lat.

Biceps femoris

Semi tend.

Semi membranosis

Linea aspera

The 'Q' Angle

NB The linea aspera is the ridge down the back of the femoral shaft from which the main powerhouse muscles arise, the shaded muscle in the diagram. The origins of these muscles are all lateral to the patella.

Fig 8 Anatomy of the thigh

Powerhouse muscles

The powerhouse muscles are the vastus lateralis, the vastus intermedius and the vastus medialis but NOT the vastus medialis oblique. (While many include the rectus femoris in the quadricep group, I believe that its function is not strictly powering extension of the knee as it crosses the hip joint, but is to do with positioning the pelvis in relation to the tibia.)

> While sitting, feet planted on the floor, try straightening the leg. The quads contract but the rectus femoris does not. Still sitting, lift the thigh. The rectus femoris contracts but the quads do not.

These power muscles pull on the kneecap to straighten the knee, their origins are attached around the top end and around the back of the femur. Thus, the direction of the pull of these muscles is up and outwards towards the outside of the hips. These thigh muscles merge into a tendon above the knee that envelops the kneecap. It is called the quadricep tendon, and it is big. The kneecap (patella) is attached by the patellar tendon to the tibia.

23

Sit with your leg out straight, your foot on a low stool and your knee unsupported and notice these things on yourself, or stand in front of a mirror. Some people with fatter thighs and knees will have to feel these things rather than see them. Possibly, use a friend's thigh to find the anatomy. When relaxed, the kneecap is loose. Move your own a bit from side to side with your fingers.

> (If your knee is sore, moving your kneecap thus is a way to gain the confidence to move and contract the muscles.)

Steering muscle

As noted, there is an angle in this 'pulley' system of quadricep muscles, patella, patellar tendon and tibia. With contraction of the quadriceps (the powerhouse muscles of the thigh), the patella is pulled upwards, but also a bit outwards. We humans have evolved a part of the thigh muscle that is attached to the inside of the kneecap exactly halfway up (3 o'clock or 9 o'clock, depending on one's point of view) and also onto the inside or medial side of the bottom third of the quadricep tendon. When this part of the muscle contracts, it pulls the kneecap inwards (medially), correcting the bowstring effect on the patella.

This will balance the pressures under the inside and outer-side facets of the patella as it moves against the femoral condyles. At the same time, it stabilises the capsule and therefore the joint, holding the bones in the right place as the joint moves.

This inward pulling muscle is called the VMO (vastus medialis oblique). It is the steering muscle (see diagrams).

Unfortunately, for people with knee pain this medial pulling part of the muscle gets lazy and weak and sometimes very difficult to find. For those with a 'good leg', try to find the muscle on the good side and then transfer to the painful side. Or use a friend's healthy leg so you can understand what it is you are looking for.

(In clinic it was often faster to use my own leg. I would see them briefly at two weeks to make sure the patient had got it right.)

Direction of pull
generated by the
powerhouse muscles,
the quadriceps

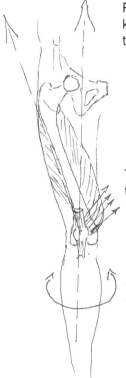

Resultant force required to straighten the
knee keeping the patella correctly aligned in
the femoral intercondylar notch

The corrective forces generated by
the VMO, the 'steering' muscle

Rotation can occur at the knee when the
foot is planted and the trunk is turned to
the left or the right. An extreme example is
shown in the Dummy Pass, Fig 5, page 19

The rotation changes the 'Q' Angle, the 'powerhouse' pulls with the
same force. The steering muscle must be constantly correcting to
keep the patella–femoral joint correctly loaded.

Fig 9 VMO correction force 2

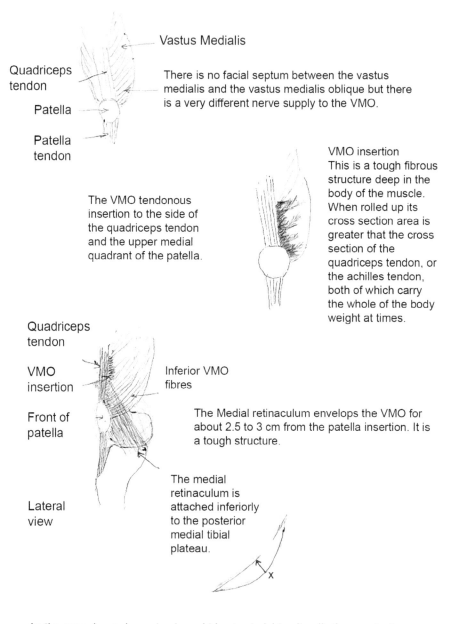

Vastus Medialis

Quadriceps
tendon

There is no facial septum between the vastus
medialis and the vastus medialis oblique but there
is a very different nerve supply to the VMO.

Patella

Patella
tendon

VMO insertion
This is a tough fibrous
structure deep in the
body of the muscle.
When rolled up its
cross section area is
greater that the cross
section of the
quadriceps tendon, or
the achilles tendon,
both of which carry
the whole of the body
weight at times.

The VMO tendonous
insertion to the side of
the quadriceps tendon
and the upper medial
quadrant of the patella.

Quadriceps
tendon

VMO
insertion

Inferior VMO
fibres

Front of
patella

The Medial retinaculum envelops the VMO for
about 2.5 to 3 cm from the patella insertion. It is
a tough structure.

The medial
retinaculum is
attached inferiorly
to the posterior
medial tibial
plateau.

Lateral
view

As the curved muscle contracts and tries to straighten it pulls the enveloping
medial retinaculum ('x' moving along the arrow up and forward) pulling the
posterior tibia forward and stabilizing the medial side of the knee. It is pulling on
the patella and therefore the lateral retinaculum and thus stabilizes the knee joint.

Fig 10 Summary of VMO anatomy and function

Biofeedback

The point of the VMO exercise is twofold:

- To improve the brain's control of that steering muscle.
- To wake up and strengthen the muscle.

Tiring any muscle is the stimulus that makes it stronger. A muscle that is tiring tries to cheat by firing off different groups of muscle fibres to spread the workload. This is called fasciculation. When doing the VMO exercise, a finger must be laid on the lowest edge of the muscle to tell the brain what is really happening, all the time! (Biofeedback)

As the muscle gets tired and starts to cheat, one can feel it and make the mental effort to drive the muscle to work harder.

(There is also room for the physio's finger beside the patient's finger.)

The nerve to this part of the VMO muscle is very special. It is huge (see Chapter 11), which means that this part of the muscle is innovated by many, many more nerve fibres than all the other muscles of the thigh. The implication is that the muscle's function is not simply power production but fine control of the application of the steering effort necessary. The VMO is a very finely controlled muscle, and all the more susceptible to the inhibitory effects of pain.

Do you need to know all this? I think it helps to understand what you are trying to do. You are trying to wake up the muscle, get the brain to relearn how to make it contract and, by making the muscle contract hard, tire or fatigue the muscle, which is the stimulus to making the muscle stronger. Better control, better strength, better function! And in particular, better care of the hyaline cartilage surfaces of the patella and the femur.

Additionally, and importantly, the action of the VMO also maintains the correct tension in the capsule and the ligaments that hold the femoral condyles on the tibia; in effect, it stabilises the knee joint (see Fig 10, page 26).

Section 3 explains the underlying science in much more detail, including the anatomy, the physiology (how the body tissues behave) and the pathology (how they misbehave).

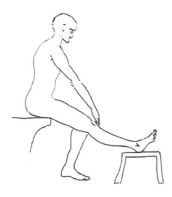

The leg is straight at the knee.
The foot points downwards and inwards,
plantar flexion or 'equinus' in the jargon.
The patient's finger rests on the lower edge of
the VMO just beside the patella to monitor the
control, Biofeedback.

There is also room for the therapist's finger.

NB There is a common fault; people sit too far
back on the chair, which results in the thigh
being slightly supported from behind and the
knee does not fall into full extension.

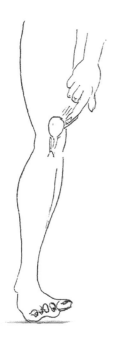

BIOFEEDBACK
To really know that the brain is controlling the
muscle the patient's finger must be on the
muscle edge throughout the exercise.

The foot is pointing downwards and inwards,
plantar flexion and inversion. This position is
brought about by the tibialis posterior deep in
the back of the calf. It is a powerful extensor
of the ankle joint.

Fig 11 Position for the isometric VMO exercise

Pure extension of the leg is best achieved sitting on the very edge of a chair, with the leg straight out, the heel supported on a low stool and unsupported at the knee. When relaxed in this position, the leg tends to roll outwards and rest on the outside of the heel, and the foot points downwards and inwards.

One common fault is that people sit too far back on the chair, such that the edge gives some support to the femur and lessens the fall of the weight of the leg into full extension at the knee.

Do not try to pull the foot up at the ankle! Do not try to raise the leg at the hip. Do not bend at the knee! (Physiotherapy has for years recommended these actions. For this exercise, forget them.)

The exercise is isometric. Isometric means that there is no movement of the knee or anything else. 'You, the mechanic, can rev the engine without moving the transmission.' Movement might trigger a stab of pain and inhibit your effort.

There might be some discomfort when contracting, but it is not a surprise. One can continue to contract the muscle and ignore the discomfort. This is important.

The index finger should be placed on the edge of the muscle, just beside the kneecap, as shown in Fig 11. Keep it there throughout the exercise, all the time! It is there so that the brain—your brain—can feel exactly what it is doing (biofeedback). The brain and the muscle must not be allowed to cheat!

> The position of the foot in plantar flexion and inversion is produced by the powerful tibialis posterior deep in the back of the calf and is often forgotten about.

The VMO Exercise

The muscle must be forced to work as hard as it can for 10 seconds, and then it is rested for 10 seconds, and then contracted again for 10 seconds, continuing on and off for two minutes—six strong contractions. It is hard work. I would say to a patient, 'If your brain can learn to control the edge of the muscle, it is controlling the rest.'

The exercise should be repeated twice a day, in a place where one is alone and can concentrate, at least until one stops going red in the face with the effort. Use the diagrams. It is further described in another chapter.

Initially, one should not do the VMO exercise as part of a general quads-strengthening exercise routine, certainly not until one is 100% confident that it is working correctly.

That is the full-blown VMO exercise. One may have to work up to it, as explained elsewhere, when recovering from the effects of the surgeon's knife, for example. I would recommend learning it before any surgical procedure of any nature on the knee, partly because you might not then need the surgery, but more so that post-op recovery of VMO function is quicker.

The VMO exercise and its application

Learning to coordinate the steering function of the quadriceps with the power function is what this book is all about. I found that it was quicker to get patients in clinic to feel my VMO if their function was poor and to look for it on their non-painful side. They could then understand what I was asking them to do. This is particularly important in patients who have completely lost the ability to contract it, and/or have rather fat thighs. However, it has always been possible, eventually, to get it to work again!

The theory behind the exercise

The exercise fatigues the muscle. This causes it to fasciculate (start to tremble). It is the muscle's normal way of sharing the work out by contracting different groups of fibres to try to spread the fatigue. This can be felt by the patient, and with concentration one can drive the whole muscle to contract. This teaches the brain to use the muscle better. The fatigue in the muscle stimulates strengthening.

It is an isometric exercise (a 'no movement' exercise). No movement means it does not trigger pain in the same way. Triggering pain is very inhibitory. It was also found that isometric exercise was more effective in the treatment of partial paralysis, such as in polio victims. Even if there is some discomfort with the contraction, contracting through the discomfort is quite possible. Even the most nervous of patients can learn to do so.

I found that if I took the time to explain to each patient why they were doing the VMO exercise and suggested that it was something they could do best when alone, most patients, particularly the adolescents with anterior knee pain, did very well. I would review my patients at two to three weeks to make sure they had understood and were really contracting the VMO, and then at six to seven weeks. Incidentally, all teenage anterior knee pain patients cured themselves within six weeks, irrespective of how many other orthopaedic surgeons and physiotherapists they had seen. Their parents, on the other hand, were sometimes rather less enamoured, possibly because they had wasted so much effort trekking around seeing other practitioners, which is why one must concentrate on teaching the patient even without the parent present.

Adults are not so used to learning new tricks, but young people are. However, adult patients, even in later life, are also capable of regaining the use of their VMO, although they may sometimes take a little longer to find the muscle.

I mentioned that my wife was teaching in a local college in Montreal and overheard these instructions being exchanged between students on a couple of occasions, which was quite pleasing.

Isometric and isotonic exercises

An isometric muscle effort is one in which there is no movement. In the era of working with acute poliomyelitis victims, where loss of muscle function was to be expected, it was observed that isometric effort was more useful than isotonic exercises at regaining some muscle function. Isotonic exercise is something like lifting a weight up and down, the same load through a range. Isometric exercise is making a continuous effort without moving, like trying to push or pull something that will just not move. In partially paralysed muscles, isometric exercise is more effective.

'Concentric loading' and 'eccentric loading' are also terms of import, but in both there is movement involved. A concentric exercise would be, for the quadricep muscle, the act of stepping up a step. The act of lowering one's weight down again is an eccentric exercise. The difference is that the muscle is contracting and shortening under load in the concentric and the muscle is lengthening under load in the eccentric. Muscles can give more work eccentrically; for example, lowering a heavy body can be controlled even if the person letting out the rope does not have the strength to pull the body up. Bodybuilders work their muscles to exhaustion concentrically and then use eccentric exercises to further fatigue the muscles they are working on.

The VMO exercise is an isometric exercise, and neither concentric nor eccentric.

I emphasise the position of leg: straight with the foot pointing down and inwards. It is important. All too often physiotherapists used to ask patients doing quadricep exercises to lift the leg up and pull the toes and the foot up and outwards towards the hip (dorsiflexion of the ankle and hip). This mixing of phases is WRONG.

The reasons it is not correct to dorsiflex the ankle, or try to lift the leg—both flexor phase actions—is that this is primarily a retraining exercise and not simply a strengthening exercise. When retraining a muscle, one must not mix extensor and flexor phases.

Practicalities

In many patients the wasting of the vastus medialis oblique is profound and there is little or no palpable function on the medial edge of the patella. In these people the first thing to do is to see if there is function on the opposite side. At the same time, I usually placed the patient's finger on my own VMO so that they could feel what I was talking about. (After a long afternoon clinic I was sometimes quite stiff the next day!)

It can take them a couple of diligent days of effort to find the muscle. Parents were sometimes a bit slow to be convinced, particularly if they had been seeing many other specialists and physiotherapists. An early follow-up visit to verify their function paid dividends and improved compliance.

Persuading my physiotherapists to do this proved surprisingly difficult. They had all been trained, it seemed, using the work of Jacqueline Perry, MD, at Ranchos Los Amigos Rehabilitation Center, who had advocated straight leg raising with weights and knee straightening with weights over a rolled-up towel, with the foot and ankle pulled up. (The many YouTube videos even now perpetuate the Dr Perry advice and error.) The first exercise is only good for strengthening the hip flexors, and the latter for strengthening the powerhouse part of the quadriceps, but they do very little or nothing for the steering effort of the VMO, and particularly not for the control of the VMO if there is any pain on movement. Dorsiflexion of the ankle only confuses the reflex control of movements.

For young people I put **absolutely no restrictions** on what they wanted to do in the way of games, sports, etc. ... and no braces or other supports.

Adults

There is always a spectrum of problems in adults. They progress from teens to young adults, and the hyaline cartilage in the patellofemoral joint matures (see section on hyaline cartilage, Chapter 13). There were a number of adult patients, mostly female, with chronic anterior knee pain and, to a greater or lesser degree, quite severe wear arthritis under the lateral facet of the patella. They were all given VMO exercises initially. Some of these patients did need surgical help. I was quite prepared to offer them an elevation and realignment operation, plus, if indicated, some sort of patelloplasty to remove any hooking osteophytes from the lateral side facet of the patella, such that it could realign medially more easily. I discuss this further on.

Older people had more difficulty waking up their VMO muscles and had to persist with their exercises for up to three months. Interestingly, most of them did. Removing their pain helps greatly their ability to rehabilitate.

Even more interesting, to me, was that muscles that were very atrophied and had not functioned for many years could be persuaded to start working again, and then worked up to normal function once the pain sources had been taken away. I rarely found reason to advance the VMO surgically.

One trick to wake up a muscle is to use a TENS machine turned up a bit as a muscle stimulator. In the remote Canadian bush the Irish physiotherapist showed me this. It makes the muscle twitch, which convinces the patient that there is something there to work on.

Return visits to clinic at two weeks to reinforce their efforts pay dividends.

This was the diagram that I would give to patients in my care.

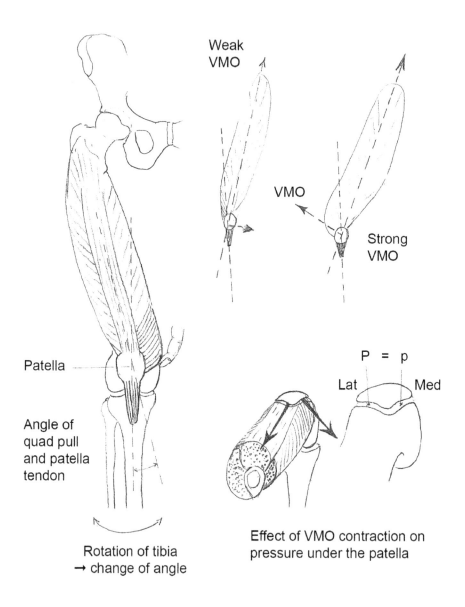

Weak VMO

VMO

Strong VMO

Patella

Angle of quad pull and patella tendon

P = p

Lat   Med

Rotation of tibia
→ change of angle

Effect of VMO contraction on pressure under the patella

Fig 12 Diagram given to patients in clinic after receiving VMO instructions

Chapter 7

Fast Track: Rehabilitation at Home

For those readers hot off the 'injury list', these are little things one can do at home to get going.

Partial weight-bearing and the bathroom scales trick

Post-op knee patients are in a bulky bandage or sometimes a cylinder cast, and foot and ankle patients tend to be in a cast or splint. At times this is with the foot pointing down (equinus). The surgeon may have stipulated 'non weight bearing' progressing to 'partial weight-bearing'.

Getting upright with crutches or a frame, rather than lying down, triggers a number of postural reflexes of which we are unaware. The person feels better even just standing with a Zimmer frame. Standing up is very beneficial to rapid recovery.

A useful trick is to rest the foot on a bathroom scales. Note what the leg plus the cast weighs with the foot effectively on the floor. For the patient, it does not feel like any load at all. It is almost always safe to put that amount of weight on the leg. Gradually, increase the weight after a few days (plus 5 kg (12 lbs)), but do not stimulate discomfort.

The order 'limited weight-bearing' is to limit the risk of damage to the repair by being impatient or overenthusiastic. Healing processes go at their own speed, and nothing we medics have done can really change the speed of the biological processes, whatever you read in the glossy magazines, and that includes hyperbaric oxygen.

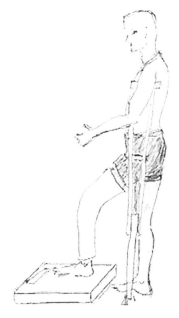

Fig 13 Bathroom scales trick: weighing the leg

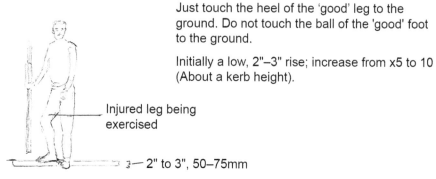

Just touch the heel of the 'good' leg to the ground. Do not touch the ball of the 'good' foot to the ground.

Initially a low, 2"–3" rise; increase from x5 to 10 (About a kerb height).

Injured leg being exercised

— 2" to 3", 50–75mm

NB Good heel touching ground, not the ball of the foot.

Progress to the bottom of a stair case, usually about 7" (185mm) and gradually increase the repetitions.

Look for a higher step to work off.

For the athlete move on to a bench, about 14" high, and then progress to two legged deep squats. Use the arms for balance bringing them forward as one goes down. For the serious skier aim at achieving 100 repetitions.

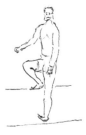

For the seriously fast man try multiple single leg squats, fast repetitions x15 on each legs at least x3 per night should clip a second off your 100m times.

Fig 14 Progressive step-up exercises

It is worth remembering that tissues sewn together actually get weaker in the early period of repair, so that 'light touch with no discomfort' may be all that is safe. Discuss this with your surgeon.

If you want as little delay to healing as possible, light touch weight-bearing and control of the swelling in the leg by elevating the leg when at rest are the most useful. Water runs downhill. Swelling delays healing, and swelling always occurs after any injury, surgical or otherwise. It is obligate (i.e. it cannot be stopped). (See remarks on inflammation and the inflammatory response, which is integral to all healing processes.)

Weight-bearing triggers all the little nervous reflexes that control the leg muscles, and also those to the blood vessels. Good circulation is very beneficial to healing. In the past we surgeons may have been a bit too conservative, but being overeager does not change the overall healing time.

Powerhouse strengthening

When necessary, introduce the powerhouse strengthening exercises with the step-up routine. As the leg improves, one seeks out higher steps so that one is dropping down and pushing up greater distances, which is working on the power function of the quads. (Fig 14 on page 36 is self-explanatory.) One cannot start this phase of rehabilitation before full weight-bearing is permitted.

For the skier or the athlete, step-ups progress to squats: deep squats on both legs, bringing the arms forwards to help balance. Work up to 100 repetitions? And for the real 'powder hound' or speedster, one leg squats: 15 times on each leg at speed, repeated three time daily.

(In my era, the French ski team all had to do one-legged squats. They were shown to me by Bobby Birrell, who held the 120 yds high-hurdle world record. One can clip about a second off one's 100 yd time!)

When to start the VMO exercise

Always start rehab of the knee with this, even pre-op. If patients can get the VMO muscle going prior to a surgical procedure, they will get going quicker post-op.

The powerhouse training can start earlier on a very low step to get going.

Step-up exercise

I recommend this as the first exercise, as it restores confidence in using the leg. It starts the strengthening in the powerhouse quadriceps (thigh muscles). I used to jokingly recommend that one could do it at a bus stop, as the curb height is only about 3 inches and one could hold onto the bus-stop pole, but please, do beware the buses![9] But the curb is about the right height to start with: a low step of 3 inches (75 mm).

The leg to be exercised stands on the step, and the heel of the good leg is lowered to the ground. One straightens the 'sick' leg, lifting the 'good' heel off the ground. If one touches the ball of the good foot to the ground, there is a strong tendency to jump or push with the good leg. This is not what this exercise is about. You are working the bad leg.

Gradually, increase the number of lifts; start with five, work up to 10, 15 even 20. Also, as you become more adept, increase the height of the lifts. Stairs are usually 7 inches (185 mm)—just a bit too high initially. Try to find something about 3 inches (75 mm).

The VMO exercise should be done during the same period, if not at the same time. It is always more important to get the steering element working before worrying too much about strengthening the powerhouse. I would often instruct the VMO exercise prior to any surgical procedure, such that they could prepare themselves at home. I never bothered about instructing hamstring exercises; they seemed to wake up as the VMO function returned.

Stationary bicycles

I personally have little experience of using them, but fellow surgeons and also surgical victims have said that they were able to get their range of motion back more easily with a stationary bicycle.

Knee surgery is painful, and anything that can relieve pain helps. It is interesting that regaining movement, either with a passive CPM (continuous passive motion) machine, sliding the foot resting on a tray on the bed or using a stationary bicycle, can significantly reduce the need for painkillers.

---

[9] And don't be stupid, like the woman who put a paper cup of coffee between her legs in a drive-through and scalded herself. She sued McDonald's for serving her hot coffee.

Elevation of the foot of the bed

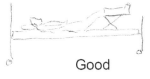

Good

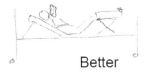

Better

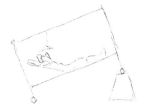

Old fashioned but BEST

With a monkey bar patients could make more physical effort to move in bed.

Remember, swelling is water and it runs downhill.

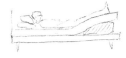

At home place the cushions off a sofa or chair under the bottom half of the mattress.

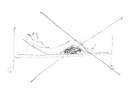

Very bad and dangerous to place pillows under the knees with the leg draped over.

It has been shown to increase the risks of pressure on the veins behind the knee and increase the risk of developing a deep veinous thrombosis.

Fig 15 Elevation of legs

Control of swelling

At home, or in hospital, it is never wrong to arrange to elevate the leg during the night, and during the day for the first five days.

Swelling is the enemy of healing. Swelling can occur below a healing injury or wound and will be worse in folk who already have a reason to swell during the day. Swelling (oedema for the purist) is essentially water that has escaped the blood vessels and escaped from within the cells into the spaces between the cells, the extra cellular space. It is called lymph. Small quantities are normal towards the end of a day spent on one's feet. But the accumulation of swelling impairs circulation, and sluggish, venous return of blood towards the heart can cause dangerous conditions, like deep venous thrombosis.

The tendency to swell is at its maximum for five days. It cannot be stopped; it is part of the healing process. Water runs downhill. For the first few days try to have the feet higher than the knees, and you knees higher than your bottom, all the time you are at rest. And, after knee surgery, rest interspersed with frequent gentle movement for these five days is quite a good thing from the healing point of view.

A pillow or cushion under the knees, so they are bent over it, may be comfortable, but it has been shown to be potentially dangerous, predisposing to Deep Venous Thrombosis (DVT); and yet in hospital one sees well-meaning nurses and physios doing it all the time.

Years ago all fractures of the lower limb were treated in bed with skeletal traction. Pull on the leg and the patient's bottom slides towards the foot of the bed. As a result, most beds in an orthopaedic ward had the foot of the bed elevated. It was almost the default position. It was called balanced traction.

When deep venous thrombosis and pulmonary embolism was being intensively investigated in the early 1970s, it was rare on the orthopaedic wards. There were cases where patients were nursed lying flat in bed for prolonged periods or put in long leg casts. Pulmonary emboli were more common on general surgical and medical wards. Persuading nursing staff to elevate the foot of a bed these days is quite difficult. They seem to know better!

Not only does elevation aid healing by reducing swelling, it reduces the risk of developing a clot (a DVT) in a deep leg vein, and that can be very dangerous. One's blood can become predisposed to clotting in a number of conditions*, one of which is the soft tissue injury of a surgical procedure. The risk increases with the immobility of recovery.

The best way to elevate the legs at home is to put cushions from the seat of a chair or sofa under the bottom half of the mattress. This way both legs are up and the affected leg does not fall off the pillow during the night.

Conscious efforts to wiggle one's toes and move one's ankles are also important.

Cautionary tales

I did have a morbidly obese youth who sustained a badly shattered proximal tibial plateau fracture while standing in the road. He was hit by a car. I did the usual: a special plate and a couple of cleverly placed screws. Imagine my horror when I met him walking on it to the toilet about 48 hours later; his arms were nothing like strong enough to take his weight with crutches. To my surprise he had an excellent result. But I still do not recommend it! I think that perhaps because he was a young male with very well-stressed, and therefore very strong, bone that held screws very well, my surgery did not fall apart.

My brother, by comparison, had an Achilles tendon repair following a rupture and at three months rode a mountain bike over a grassy field and re-ruptured his tendon. A further three months of complete splintage and three more months of being very careful were needed!

*Causes of predisposition to DVT
1. Soft tissue injury;
2. Immobility with the legs horizontal or down (e.g. air travel);
3. Dehydration;
4. Contraceptive pills (the older ones);
5. Pregnancy;
6. Cancer;
7. Age;
8. Obesity;
9. Smoking;
10. Heart failure;
11. Inflammatory renal diseases;
12. Genetic predisposition.

SECTION 3

The Science

'I know well that the reader has no great desire to know all this, but I have the desire to tell them of it.'

Jean Jacques Rousseau

———•◦•———

Now, perhaps I can interest you in the science behind my recommendations for rehabilitation of the knee. Understanding what one is trying to achieve can make achieving it much easier.

And some are quite keen to know what it is all about.

(For a lay person reading this book, a practical suggestion might be that you skip this until you have read the later sections.)

Chapter 8

Application of Basic Science: Anatomy, Physiology and Pathology

Physiology is basically how the body tissues are supposed to work. Pathology is broadly how it goes wrong. Anatomy is … anatomy, **the parts involved**. This, in one's thinking, should include the cells involved. Claude Bernard's '*le milieu intèrieur*' tends to get overlooked. (It also has a new name, 'Homeostasis', which does not actually impart the same meaning.)

The *milieu intèrieur* is the idea that each cell is living in its own little environment. Each cell's metabolism requires quite specific conditions, which differ for different tissues; for example, oxygen concentration is high in the tissues of the lungs and high in the brain but very low in the depth of hyaline cartilage. Osteocytes and chondrocytes (the basic cells of bone and cartilage) live in this low-oxygen environment; their metabolism is probably very slow, unless stimulated in some way. They respond to physical strains or stresses, probably in response to piezoelectric currents triggered by strain in the calcium apatite crystals and the collagen fibres under load. Lack of stresses in prolonged space travel causes very significant loss of calcium from the bones. This also occurs in chronically bed bound patients. These cells are evidently alive and doing something, even if it is done slowly.

Ultimately, diffusion of molecules through the extra cellular fluid—fluid that is outside the cell wall and outside the lumen (the inside space) of blood vessels—is the mechanism of exchange everywhere in the body of everything: oxygen, carbon dioxide, glucose, sodium, potassium and any other chemical, such as hormones, antibiotics or other drugs. The transport of oxygen, nourishments and metabolites is good where there is good blood circulation and slower where circulation is poor, or where there is no blood supply. Under these conditions, cells have to rely on diffusion of molecules through the fluid of the intercellular spaces for relatively longer distances, which is of course much slower.

In the case of chondrocytes in hyaline articular cartilage, the cartilage is like a firm sponge, when squeezed under load and movement the fluid in it is squeezed out. As the load is lessened, the joint fluid is pulled back into the matrix of the cartilage, probably by the electrical charges on the proteins, which are all negative and mutually repel each other, trying to spring apart. This microscopic circulation of joint fluid is the only nourishment that cartilage cells get to maintain the structure and attempt to repair it. Yes, I believe that there is a potential for cartilage repair if one gets the exact conditions right for the chondrocyte metabolism.

Failure to consider the perfect conditions for the cells one is trying to help is a big factor in the failure of some therapies. There was a concept of 'The Sick Cell Syndrome', which, like so many things in medicine, has come into and out of and back into fashion over the last 50 years. The practical application is: **when in doubt, try to do the things that would make for the ideal conditions for the cells of the organ you are treating**. A very real example of this is the concept of 'early movement' in modern orthopaedic surgery.

Movement

Who, or what, you should ask, are you trying to move? It would be more pertinent to ask, what is movement? How much? How far? For cells like osteocytes and chondrocytes, a few microns of movement is colossal; they are only 10μ or 15μ in diameter. They respond to just a very little movement. The modern vogue for requiring visible ranges of motion and total reliance on internal fixations is, I think, overkill. From the cellular point of view, one can achieve significant movement within a cast or splint that can aid healing, particularly with partial weight-bearing in the case of a leg.

I used a padded POP (plaster of Paris) splint for ankle fracture surgery followed at about three weeks by the removal of sutures and the application of a walking cast, fully weight-bearing, for about seven to eight weeks. When this was removed, patients did not need physiotherapy. There was enough micro-movement in the cast for good healing and muscle recovery to occur.

Swelling and the acute inflammatory response

Note that inflammation is the only response that all tissues of the body can make to any trauma: thermal, mechanical, chemical—one response. The understanding of the inflammatory response is important when treating injured tissues.

The initial five days following injury involves an immediate histamine release that causes the tiny pores between the cells forming the walls of the capillary blood vessels (the podocytes) to become bigger, and the vessels start to leak. One cannot stop this. The mineral solution, along with the proteins, white blood cells, lymphocytes, neutrophils and monocytes, can escape from inside the capillaries and start the process of swelling. Healing involves the palisading and differentiating of white cells into fibroblasts, the cleaning up and removal of dead tissue and any bacteria and gradually laying down new collagen repair tissue.

Normally, the bigger molecules, in particular albumin (64,430 mol. wt. cf. water (H_2O) at 18 mol. wt.), cannot escape from the vessel lumen and by the process of osmosis draw or hold the fluid within the lumen of the blood vessels. Osmosis, you may remember, is dependent upon the number of molecules in a solution, not the size of the molecules. Once these large molecules are out in the fluid between the cells, the albumin, and any other molecules, start to draw more fluid in the other direction out of the lumen of the blood vessels. This we recognise as swelling. In soft tissues one can press it with one's finger and leave a dent. It stiffens the tissues and tends to restrict the flow of venous blood and lymph.

However, in bone the consequences are very different. Bone forms a rigid box around all the soft tissue structures, like the blood vessels. Very quickly, the formation of oedema causes the pressure to rise above the venous drainage pressure and then exceeds the arterial inflow pressure. The bone becomes **ischaemic** (no blood flow and no oxygen) locally for at least 1 cm from a fracture line or from a drill hole for a fixation screw. This would not seem to be the ideal situation to get a circulating antibiotic into the area, nor for the health of the cells involved in the healing process.

Ultimately, diffusion of molecules is the mechanism of exchange everywhere in the body of everything: oxygen, carbon dioxide, glucose, electrolytes, waste metabolite and any other chemical, such as an antibiotic or other drugs. Fortunately, osteocytes and chondrocytes seem to have a very slow metabolism and seem to be more resistant to these unfavourable conditions.

Osmosis

Osmosis is the obligatory movement of fluid molecules from a low concentration solution into a higher concentration solution when they are separated by a semi-permeable membrane, one that permits the passage of the solvent molecules but not the passage of the dissolved molecules. Osmosis has nothing to do with the size of the molecules, only the relative numbers of molecules. Molecular weight is a reflection of the number of atoms that make up a molecule of anything.

Elevation

Another little 'rocking horse' of mine is elevation of the limb, preferably by elevating the foot of the bed. Part of the reasoning is as above: it helps reduce the swelling locally to the injury, and swelling delays healing. As importantly in lower limb injury, where there is risk of immobility, it reduces the risks of developing a deep venous thrombosis, which is the precursor to the potentially fatal condition of a pulmonary embolus[10].

To my knowledge there was only one useful paper in the whole medical literature on comparing elevation of the foot of the bed (i.e. the legs) to any of the other modalities of management of the risks of DVT (deep venous thrombosis) formation. (There are thousands of papers on DVT prevention with drugs, elastic stockings, pressure pumps and other expensive mechanical toys.) The paper I recall compared the elevation of the foot of the operating table at 15–30 degrees (ankles higher than knees higher than buttocks, known as the Trendelenburg position) to the use of a mechanical apparatus that moved the ankle joints continuously during the operation. It clanked and was a bit irritating (circa 1970). The belief was that the complete immobility of the patient on the operating table, coupled with the traumatic physiological stress of surgery—which predisposed to the clotting of blood in the venous lakes of the calf muscles and can lead to the formation of DVT in the leg veins—would be lessened by elevation and could prevent the stasis.

Detecting the presence of an early DVT in those days was done with radioactive labelled fibrinogen (I_{131}), and it could be detected in the calf muscles with a Geiger counter. It was very sensitive and clearly demonstrated that elevation of the foot of the table at 10 degrees was more effective than the mechanical thing and elasticated bandages. It also made us realise that DVT occurred just as dangerously in the non-damaged leg in someone in bed—the so called 'silent limb'.

(One consequence of that work is the habit of resting the Achilles tendons on a sandbag to let the calf muscles hang loose when a patient is on the operating table, and another is the use of below-knee, elasticated 'anti-embolic' stockings.)

---

[10] **Causes of predisposition to DVT**
1. Soft tissue injury; 2. Immobility with the legs horizontal or down (e.g. air travel);
3. Dehydration: 4. The pill (the older ones); 5. Pregnancy; 6. Cancer; 7. Age; 8. Obesity;
9. Smoking; 10. Heart failure; 11. Inflammatory renal diseases; 12. Genetic predisposition.

Virchow, in 1856, made three postulates predisposing to DVT formation:

- 'Intrinsic' changes in the chemistry of the blood, making it more likely to clot (the stress of trauma or surgery, the presence of cancer, pregnancy, smoking, dehydration, inflammatory bowel disease, heart failure, age—the list is depressingly quite long).
- 'Extrinsic' changes, by which he meant damage to the blood vessel walls.
- 'Stasis', or lack of drainage (lying in bed, prolonged sitting (air travel), prolonged lying on the operating table).

In the early 1970s almost all lower-limb fractures in the UK were treated in bed with traction for up to three months. Balanced traction meant lifting the foot of the bed up to stop the patient's bottom sliding towards the foot of the bed when one pulled on the limb. It is actually a comfortable position if one wishes to sit up in bed. It also ensures drainage in the lower limbs. DVT and pulmonary embolus were not really orthopaedic problems, except in people in long leg casts and lying in bed after spinal surgery, or those who had been operated on for fixation. Almost everybody else had the foot of their beds raised. It was the default position.

This was in contrast to the incidence of DVT and, sadly, pulmonary embolus on general surgical and gynaecology wards and the medical wards, where the beds were mostly flat.

Elevation of the foot of your bed costs nothing, is comfortable and is safe. At home, following discharge from hospital, the best manner to achieve this is to place the seat cushions from a sofa or armchair under the mattress. If the leg is simply elevated on pillows, it always falls off as the patient moves or sleeps (see Fig 15, page 39).

Swelling slows healing

The simple treatment of swollen ankles due to the build-up of fluid is to rest the leg elevated. Elevated means that the ankle is higher than the knee, which is higher than the bottom! Lying with the leg over a pillow (beloved of nurses and physiotherapists, I am sad to say) is not elevation. It is dangerous, as it slows the return of blood from the foot, ankle and calf by pressing on the veins at the back of the knee. The risk is the formation of a deep venous thrombosis, and if that breaks away, it will cause a pulmonary embolus and can easily lead to death. Sadly, it was a constant war over the years to get patients nursed with their legs correctly elevated. It is actually more comfortable to lie with the legs a little elevated when sitting in bed; one's bottom does not tend to slide down the bed away from the backrest.

Lay reader, I belabour this point about elevation because it is your life that is being put at risk. Once you are home, whatever advice you have been given, you can do no harm by resting with your leg elevated, preferably both legs. The simplest way at home is to place the thick cushions from the seat of a sofa or armchair under the bottom half of the mattress. The legs are up and drain, and they do not fall off the advised pillows.

In the inflammatory response, the lymphocytes (a type of white cell) also escape out of the blood vessels and seem to trigger the appearance of fibroblasts that palisade (i.e. line up) and turn into fibrocytes, which start to organise the healing process of the soft tissues. As a surgeon, and as a patient, one wants the soft tissue envelope to seal off the fracture site or the repair from the risks of bacteria as quickly as possible.

After five or six days, in my practice, the patient could hop around letting the ball of the foot touch the ground. The useful trick is to get the patient to rest their foot on a bathroom scales (Fig 13, page 35) to the point of a couple of stone (15 kg).

Try it. It feels like nothing. By touching the ball of the foot to the floor, there is reflex neurological feedback to the normal muscles of walking. There may not be much visible movement to the eye of the observer, but from the point of view of the osteocytes, chondrocytes and fibroblasts, there is plenty of movement.

(This practice evolved in the remote north-west of British Columbia, where physiotherapy was very limited and distances were impractical for patients. Their recovery was as good, if not better, than urban populations dutifully attending their local physiotherapy departments.)

I had a workman's compensation patient who refused to walk on his injured leg and was 'suffering' excruciating pain and had to use crutches! He fell and broke his other ankle, which needed a cast. He also needed to get to the bathroom, regularly! Immediately, his compensation leg healed completely!

Tissue strength post-repair

An important effect of the inflammatory response is that initially it causes the damaged and repaired tissues to weaken, so that repairs are actually at their weakest at 14 days post-op, and gradually over the next 14 to 20 days the tissues begin to strengthen. 'How long before I can…?' For most repairs it is at least 21 to 28 days before anything gets stronger. Hence, the magic six weeks of 'Be very careful', and often 12 weeks or more. The use of hyperbaric oxygen and various medicines cannot and do not speed the processes of repair.

(Achilles tendon rupture patients, be even more careful because 16 to 20 weeks post-injury and one can still re-rupture! As did my brother!)

Plaster of Paris casts

POP is very 'hi-tech' compared with fibreglass. It draws off any moisture from the wound, it is a very good wound dressing (it was previously used for the management of varicose ulcers), it gradually softens and gently increases the range of movement, and with fierce injunction from the surgeon to keep the cast clean and dry, it ensures better compliance from many a patient.

> (A completely useless titbit of information: in the 1980s in New York there were two choices for the immobilisation of the cervical spine in the case of a fracture or ligament damage. One was a modern halo frame screwed to the patient's skull and a plastic vest to which it was attached by carbon-fibre rods. The other was an old-fashioned plaster of Paris minerva cast. The latter had much better patient compliance because the patients' companions would remove the halos and vests and try to sell them to another hospital!)

Chapter 9

Anatomy of the Leg Bones and the Angles Involved

'Think of the parts involved.'

I was privileged to be taught by an elderly Canadian thoracic surgeon with a propensity to confound we students by putting up chest X-rays with ambiguous shadows and asking for sensible comments. The 'parts' in his case were skin, breast tissue, underlying muscle, bone, pleura, parenchyma, bronchi, heart, blood vessels, etc., all of which would be superimposed on a chest film. This principle of thinking of the parts involved needs to be applied even unto the smallest items, right down to the cellular level if one really wants to understand the body, and particularly to the joints.

Anatomy seems to be a stumbling block for so many people in medicine. It was thrust at them while they were medical students eager to get on with the 'important' business of diagnosis and treatment of 'real' patients. To their chagrin, upon reviewing their curriculum on day one, there were months of boring, basic sciences 'far, far from' patients (in clinic it does sometimes feel like 'the maddening crowds'). The most daunting and time-consuming portion of this schedule appeared to be anatomy. To make it worse, it is often poorly taught and often without apparent reference to diseases. It is something that just had to be learned by rote.

To a large extent, the basis of this book is based on an appreciation of anatomy, both macro and microscopic. I make no excuse for belabouring it but will try to describe it from a functional point of view as quickly as is possible. To this end, I am forever indebted to Jack Laste, FRCS, one of the grand old men of learning at the Royal College of Surgeons to whose book on surgical anatomy I would still refer anyone who is having difficulty with the subject. He makes mention of the size of the nerve to the VMO.

I apologise to the lay reader if I slip into medical terms like 'varus' and 'valgus' without explanation, but it is so second nature to an orthopod or physiotherapist; it refers to the alignment of the distal part in relation to the proximal part (i.e. does it point outwards (lateral) or inwards (medial) when looked at from the front?). Valgus and lateral are the same thing; both have an 'L' in the word if that helps. A valgus knee is knock-kneed and a varus knee is a bow-legged. Other jargon words to note are 'proximal' and 'distal', e.g the foot is distal to the ankle or the proximal end of the femur is at the hip joint; 'medial' and 'lateral' are the side toward the mid line and the side away from the mid line.

Varus is the more distal part angling inwards toward the mid line. Bowed legs are in varus. In valgus the distal part angles away from the mid line, hence valgus knees are 'knock knees'.

VARUS KNEES   VALGUS KNEES
'Bow' legs   'Knock' knees

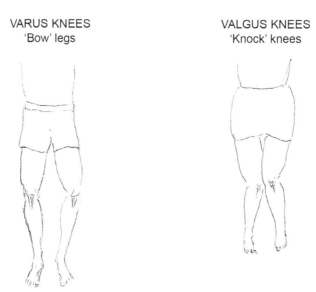

Note that the patella tendon almost aligns with the powerhouse muscles and therefore the VMO tends to do less work and to be smaller.

The powerhouse muscles and the patella tendon form a higher 'Q' Angle. The pulley system needs much more VMO corrective effort.

Fig 16 The meaning of 'varus' and 'valgus'

Bones and understanding the angles

1. The hips are apart, the knees and ankles are together. This creates an angle between the axes of the femoral shaft and the tibial shafts. This is the **Carrying Angle**. See Fig 1, page 16.

2. There is a gender difference: the female hip joints are further apart than the male's. The female femoral neck is shorter and the female femoral head is of smaller relative diameter. This all results in the angle of the femoral shaft to the tibial shaft, looked at from the front, being greater in women. This is the **Carrying Angle** and is **fixed** for each individual (not to be confused with the **'Q' Angle**, which is very **changeable** (see below)).

3. The line of weight-bearing down a leg is from the centre of the femoral head to the heel pad that is in contact with the ground. When draw in, the line ideally passes through the middle of the knee, the tibial spines. However, in perfectly normal individuals it may fall more medially onto the medial femoral condyles or even completely medial to the medial condyles, a situation known as a **varus knee** (bow-legged), or to the lateral side of the knee, resulting in a **valgus knee** (knock-kneed). The 'normal' weight distribution during walking is about 60/40 medial to lateral, as we do not completely move our weight over the bearing leg as we walk, unless it is a slow march. This is why we can trip up so easily if we catch our foot in mid stride.

4. The **valgus knee** (knocked-knee) tends to be a female configuration because of the higher Carrying Angle. It appears to be accentuated with the accumulation of fat on the insides of the thighs. Although these are 'normal' variations, they have profound implications for the loading in the medial and lateral compartments of the knee joint and in the loading of the patellofemoral joint between the kneecap and the femoral condyles.[11]

5. I draw your attention to the position of the tibial tubercle. The patellar tendon is attached to this point, and therefore all the power of the quadricep muscles extending the knee via the patella is directed to this point when the leg is being straightened.

6. Compartments? The knee is, in effect, three joints in the same sack of fluid. The medial femoral and tibial condyles articulate, the lateral femoral and tibial condyles articulate and the patella (kneecap) articulates with the upper, central part of the femoral condyle and the two sides of the intercondylar femoral notch. There is no overlap between each of these pairs of weight-bearing surfaces but they do share the same synovial fluid, so any chemical change in the fluid affects all the compartments.

---

[11] I had a grossly obese man in Canada who came to me with pain in his lateral compartments of his knees. His grossly fat thighs made him appear to have valgus knees. Years later I saw him again, very much reduced in weight and, in reality, with mildly bowed legs and now with pain in his medial compartments from overload and early osteoarthritis developing.

7. Note the position of the anterior superior iliac spine (ASIS). It is a reference point for we medics because one can always find it to feel, even if one has to dig a little bit.

The 'Q' Angle

The 'Q' Angle is the angle between the line from the ASIS to the midpoint of the patella, and from there to the tibial tubercle.

It is a mobile concept in that it changes greatly during active and passive movements of the hips, the knees and the subtalar joints under the ankle. It also varies as we turn left or right off a planted foot. There is not only bending and extending of the knee; in humans there is rotation of the femur on the tibia.

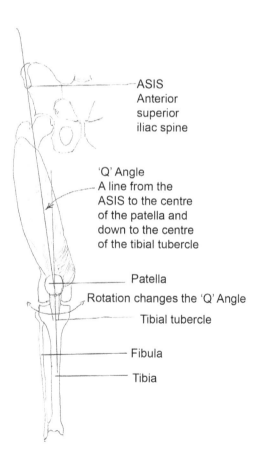

Fig 17 To illustrate the 'Q' Angle

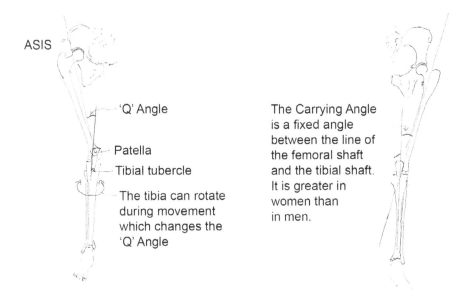

ASIS

'Q' Angle

Patella

Tibial tubercle

The tibia can rotate
during movement
which changes the
'Q' Angle

The Carrying Angle
is a fixed angle
between the line of
the femoral shaft
and the tibial shaft.
It is greater in
women than
in men.

Fig 18 Contrast the 'Q' Angle and the Carrying Angle

Explore these things on yourself:

1. Sit on a chair with the knees bent at 90 degrees, the foot flat on the floor. Rock the foot from its medial side to its lateral side (inversion and eversion). This movement takes place at the sub-talar joint and causes the tibia to rotate. This changes the 'Q' Angle. It can be a problem for long-distance runners.

2. Still sitting, knee at 90 degrees, point the foot inwards and then outwards; the rotation takes place at the knee, changing the 'Q' Angle, brought about by the hamstring muscles.

3. Flexion and extension of the hip, as in walking or running, causes the pelvis to rotate on the femur. Look at the exaggerated action of racing walkers as they rotate their pelvis forwards with each stride. This also causes the 'Q' Angle to change.

4. Sit on the edge of a chair with the leg out straight, resting the outside of the heel on a low stool. The knee straightens and the tibia rolls a little outwards in relation to the femur. This changes the 'Q' Angle. To flex the knee from this position requires the 'Q' Angle to be reduced BEFORE any flexion can occur. Note that this rotation of the tibia on the femur is limited by the cruciate ligaments which wind up against each other and have to unwind slightly to permit the knee to bend.

If standing in this position, knee locked straight, on the ski hill or rugby pitch and someone hits your knee hard causing it to bend suddenly without enough time to derotate a little, the anterior cruciate ligament can rupture! It can do so on landing from a 'spike' jump in basketball.

(One should always stand with the knees a little flexed. It might look funny, but it is safer for the knees. Standing and walking on high heels keeps the knees a little bent, and for some women all that they need to live with ACL ruptures is slightly raised heels.)

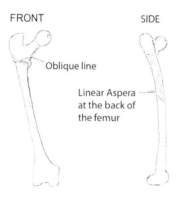

FRONT   SIDE

Oblique line

Linear Aspera at the back of the femur

The muscles are only attached to the proximal one third as they have to slide over the distal femur with flexion of the knee.

Fig 19 Quads attachment to femur

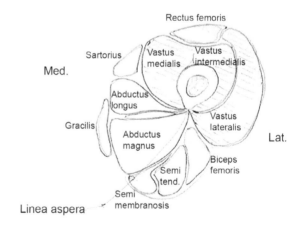

Rectus femoris

Sartorius

Vastus medialis

Vastus intermedialis

Med.

Abductus longus

Gracilis

Abductus magnus

Vastus lateralis

Lat.

Biceps femoris

Semi tend.

Semi membranosis

Linea aspera

NB The linea aspera is the ridge down the back of the femoral shaft from which the main powerhouse muscles arise, the shaded muscle in the diagram. The origins of these muscles are all lateral to the patella.

Fig 20 Anatomy of the thigh

Chapter 10

Anatomy of the Quadricep Muscles and the Vastus Medialis Oblique

There are those who deny that the vastus medialis oblique is a separate muscle from the vastus medialis. I believe they are wrong. I agree that there is no clear fascial separation, but there is a very different nerve supply to the distal vastus medialis, which I believe defines the vastus medialis oblique as functionally different. That nerve cannot be denied. It was pointed out by Jack Laste, FRCS, in his book on surgical anatomy. I describe it below.

There are two distinct functions required of the muscles of the thigh. One, which appears obvious, is to straighten the knee and move the body's weight around; I have called them the **powerhouse** muscles. The other function is **steering** which is the function of the vastus medialis oblique. The steering functions are more subtle. They are as follows:

- To steer the patella in the patellofemoral groove.
- To equalise the pressures under the medial and lateral facets of the patella.
- To maintain tension in the medial patellar retinaculum.
- To maintain tension in the lateral patellar retinaculum.
- The medial and lateral retinacula attach towards the back of the top end of the tibia and when tightened pull it forwards under the femur, and thus:
- To stabilise the femoral condyles on the tibial plateau.

A further function of some of the thigh musculature seems to be to **stabilise** the quadricep mass so there is no uncontrolled variation or wobble in the direction of application of the force produced by the powerhouse quads on the patellofemoral articulation.

Stabilisation of the power muscles seems to be the function of the tensor fascia lata and the iliotibial tract and possibly also sartorius, reasoned from the need and the alignment of the muscles and their attachments.

The powerhouse muscles

These are the vastus lateralis, the vastus medialis and the vastus intermedius. **I do not include the rectus femoris nor the Vastus Medialis Oblique**.

Note that the quadricep power muscles are all attached proximally on the femur, some at the front, some at the side and some at the back (the linea aspera). The muscles are not attached below the upper third of the femoral shaft, as the whole mass of the quadriceps needs to be able to slide over the bone as the knee bends and straightens. Note also that the power muscles' origins are all lateral to the patella and the patellar tendon and so create a 'bow string' effect in the pulley system (see Fig 19, page 56).

After a severe fracture of the distal femoral shaft, the muscles sometimes become adherent to the bone and prevent flexion of the knee. A surgical lysis of the adhesions is occasionally required to regain the range of movement. (NB to surgeons: if one uses CPM immediately post-op for a few sessions daily for four or five days, the patients will retain the movement gained, but if the limb is stabilised with dressings, one risks reformation of the adhesions.)

The overall size of the quadriceps is a reflection of the work these muscles, both the powerhouse and steering muscles, have to do. The 112 lb teenager grows into the 220 lb adult. The powerhouse muscles that have to lever that weight out of the chair or off the loo therefore get proportionally very much stronger as we get heavier. The steering element may or may not keep up. And that is the root cause of so many knee problems. Similarly, the tendons transmitting the forces also get very much thicker (discussed below in the text).

These power muscles merge into a common tendon, the quadricep tendon, which attaches to, or envelops, the patella. The tendon continues as the patellar tendon to the tibial tubercle to complete the pulley system[12].

---

[12] It can also can pull off from the top of the patella; so-called 'rupture of the quadriceps' is more often avulsion of the tendon from the bone. I can assure you that it hurts and is not to be recommended.

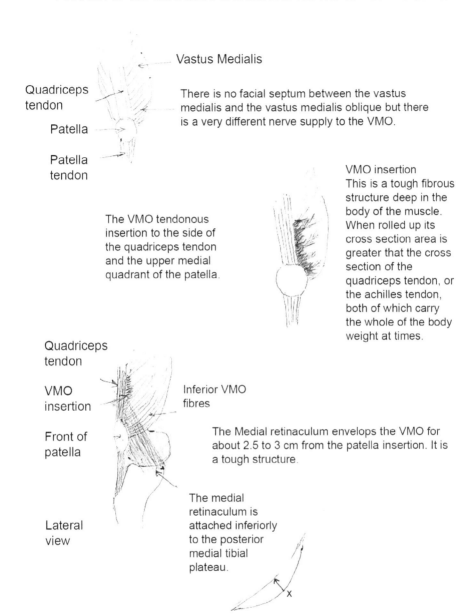

Vastus Medialis

Quadriceps tendon

There is no facial septum between the vastus medialis and the vastus medialis oblique but there is a very different nerve supply to the VMO.

Patella

Patella tendon

VMO insertion
This is a tough fibrous structure deep in the body of the muscle. When rolled up its cross section area is greater that the cross section of the quadriceps tendon, or the achilles tendon, both of which carry the whole of the body weight at times.

The VMO tendonous insertion to the side of the quadriceps tendon and the upper medial quadrant of the patella.

Quadriceps tendon

VMO insertion

Inferior VMO fibres

Front of patella

The Medial retinaculum envelops the VMO for about 2.5 to 3 cm from the patella insertion. It is a tough structure.

Lateral view

The medial retinaculum is attached inferiorly to the posterior medial tibial plateau.

As the curved muscle contracts and tries to straighten it pulls the enveloping medial retinaculum ('x' moving along the arrow up and forward) pulling the posterior tibia forward and stabilizing the medial side of the knee. It is pulling on the patella and therefore the lateral retinaculum and thus stabilizes the knee joint.

Fig 21 VMO anatomy and function as stabiliser of the knee

The steering muscle

This is the vastus medialis oblique (VMO). It is the most important muscle to understand when discussing the knee. In steering the patella, it maintains the tension in the anteromedial capsule and the anterolateral capsule (the retinacula), thereby very much helping to stabilise the femur on the tibia during movement.

(NB There is a lot of information on Fig 21; take your time to study and understand it, particularly how the VMO can tighten the medial retinaculum.)

Just as important is the VMO's role in maintaining the correct pressure between the hyaline surfaces in the patellofemoral joint for good cartilage nutrition.

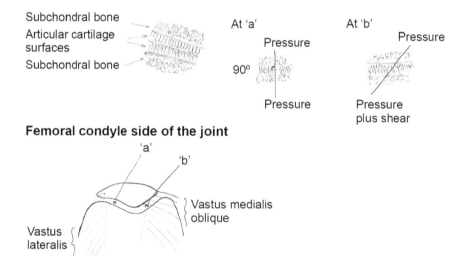

Fig 22 Pressure and shear at the joint between the patella and the femur

The VMO has a very different nerve supply compared to the other quadricep muscles. The nerve is a very much thicker one than the nerves to the rest of the muscles in the thigh. It can always be dissected out up to the inguinal ligament. It may be accompanied by the nerves to the vastus medialis and even branches to the rectus femoris, but they can always be dissected off from the nerve to the VMO.

It is, for example, much larger than the median nerve at the wrist. Jack Laste, FRCS, pointed this out 60 years ago, but its functional significance seemed to get lost.

The implications of the big nerve are that the motor units of the VMO muscle are orders of magnitude smaller than the motor units of the rest of the thigh muscles. In that case, it would be more susceptible to the inhibitory effects of pain. (Motor units are discussed in Chapter 11 under Nerve Supply to the Quadriceps (page 66).)

The majority of the quadriceps are innovated from L3, L4 and L5. By contrast, the large nerve to the VMO comes from L1 and L2 (i.e. from higher in the spinal column).

Insertion of the steering muscle
(See Fig 21)

The VMO muscle is on the medial side of the quadriceps group. It is contiguous with and below the vastus medialis; there is no fascial separation, as discussed above. The origin of the VMO's fibres are from the medial side of the linea aspera and the fascia over the adductors. The upper fibres angle down at about 45 degrees parallel to the vastus medialis fibres. The insertion of these angled fibres is to the medial side of the quadriceps tendon. The lower fibres of the VMO are almost horizontal. Their insertions are onto the upper medial quadrant of the patella itself. As the VMO contracts, it tightens both medial and lateral retinacula, as well as equalising the pressures under the patella.

The insertion of the VMO is thick tendonous tissue that arises deep in the muscle belly as a sort of fanlike structure. When dissected out and rolled up its cross-sectional area is significantly greater than the cross-sectional area of the Achilles tendon, a tendon that carries all our weight, or the patellar tendon. The evolution of this thick structure would suggest that it has a powerful job to perform. We humans are the only creatures to have evolved the VMO muscle.[13]

---

[13] Interestingly, chimpanzees and the other apes do not have a vastus medialis oblique. They do not need one. Nor do the quadrupeds, wherein the knee joint is very much a hinge with no rotation. There was a dreadful knee prosthesis called a Sheehan, which looked a bit like a sheep's knee. It did not really permit rotation until the fixing cement in the tibia gave way. I had the pleasure of replacing a fair number of them.

Insertion of the powerhouse quadriceps

The powerhouse muscles merge into one tendon—the quadricep tendon—that attaches to the top, proximal pole, of the patella. In effect, the tendon envelops the bone. The power from all these muscles, with the notable exception of the VMO, is directed through the patellar tendon, which attaches the lower pole of the patella to the tibial tubercle. When they pull, the knee is pulled straight.

Other quadricep thigh muscles

Rectus femoris

The rectus femoris (RF) also inserts into the same place on the proximal pole of the patella, and so acts through it, pulling on the patellar tendon attached to the tibial tubercle. The RF is a little different in function, in that its effort crosses both the knee and the hip joints. Its function is possibly more about balancing the attitude or alignment of the pelvis on the top of the femur, or it might be generating a Starling Law effect for the quads, in that it is being stretched as the hip extends, and so it might be triggering the extension effort of the quads to straighten the knee when running hard.

Rectus femoris has two origins. One is arcuate and fascial around the hip capsule, and the other is onto the anterior inferior iliac spine. RF muscle fibres merge into a short tendon that merges with the quadricep tendon at the proximal patellar pole.

If one sits square on a chair with the knees at 90 degrees of flexion and tries to lift the leg, the rectus femoris contracts, but not the rest of the quads. If, in that sitting position, one tries to straighten the knee against the planted foot, the quads contract but the rectus femoris does not. This suggests that it might function as part of flexor phase rather than extensor phase.

Articularis genu

Articularis genu is another functionally separate quadricep muscle. It is the deepest part of the intermedius and inserts onto the top end of the synovial sack or joint capsule. It retracts the synovial sack upwards during extension of the knee, so that it does not get pinched in the patellofemoral joint.

There is a rather uncertain test that some people do when examining the knee: they weigh heavily on the top of the patella and ask the patient to contract their quads. Yes, it hurts. But what does it show? That the examiner is trying to inflict pain? I see no value in it as a clinical sign at all.

Medial retinaculum

(See Fig 21)

The fascia over the distal and inferior fibres of the VMO muscle is quite a thick structure (*it takes sutures very well*) and the fibres cross the direction of muscle fibres at 90 degrees. It is part of the medial capsule of the knee joint and is the medial retinaculum.

Distally, it inserts with the joint capsule towards the back of the tibial plateau.

When one is opening the medial side of the knee joint with a sub-vastus incision, one cuts up beside the quadricep tendon through fairly thin capsular material, which thickens a little proximally, and then, as the incision turns medially and backwards just below and parallel to the inferior fibres of VMO at the midpoint of the medial side of the patella, it is through quite a thick band of fascial, tendon-like tissue for about 2.5–3 cm when suddenly there is again nothing but the inferior fibres of the muscle and some flimsy connective tissue. This thickened band is a very definite structure, and therefore has a function. It takes sutures well during wound closure. I always called it the medial retinaculum. It is attached to the tibia inferiorly towards the back of the medial plateau.

The functional significance of this thickening is related to the curve of the muscle fibres (see Fig 21, bottom). As the VMO muscle contracts its fibres to try to become straight, it pulls its fascial capsule, which is intimate with the joint capsule, up, pulling the posteromedial corner of the tibial plateau forwards under the femur.

Because the VMO is also pulling the patella medially in the femoral groove, it is tensioning the lateral retinaculum of the joint capsule, which tightens up the lateral capsule and tends to pull the posterolateral corner of the tibial plateau forwards.

In effect, the femur is held on the top of the tibia by a capsular/tendinous hood, which is dynamically stabilised by the VMO.

In pulling the patella onto its medial articular surface, the VMO increases the pressure under the medial articular facets and relieves some of the pressure under the lateral facets of the patella. The same mechanism also lessens the possibility of shear on the medial facets of the patella (see Figs 22, page 60 and even Fig 12, page 34). In this way it ensures the health of the articular hyaline cartilage.

Understanding this is important in treating anterior patellofemoral knee pain, whether it is spontaneous, as in the adolescent or middle-aged female, or as a result of a surgical procedure. In all cases they need emphasis on retraining the VMO.

Hamstrings

I have said nothing about the hamstring muscles, which are behind the thigh, arising from the pelvis and inserting onto the tibia. Their functions are primarily to flex, or bend, the knee. By pulling on one or other side, they rotate the tibia under the femoral condyles. However, in my practice I did not dwell on their rehabilitation, because once any injury to them had healed, and providing that the VMO function was re-established correctly, they just seemed to fall into line.

I do not deny that they need to be warmed up and stretched occasionally prior to energetic use, but as far as being the causes or the solution to pain in the knee. In my opinion, I do not think they play a significant role in knee pain and the rehabilitation thereof.

Chapter 11

Nerve Supply to the Quadriceps

'Is this important?' you ask. 'Yes, very,' is my reply. And hence I trial you with it.

The implications of the difference in size between the relatively small nerves to the power muscles of the thigh and the huge nerve to the distal medialis muscle is key to understanding the knee.

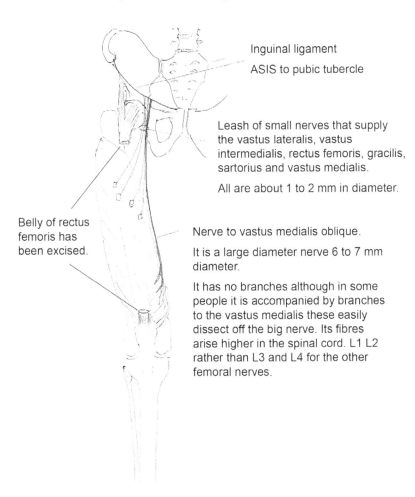

Inguinal ligament
ASIS to pubic tubercle

Leash of small nerves that supply the vastus lateralis, vastus intermedialis, rectus femoris, gracilis, sartorius and vastus medialis.

All are about 1 to 2 mm in diameter.

Belly of rectus femoris has been excised.

Nerve to vastus medialis oblique.

It is a large diameter nerve 6 to 7 mm diameter.

It has no branches although in some people it is accompanied by branches to the vastus medialis these easily dissect off the big nerve. Its fibres arise higher in the spinal cord. L1 L2 rather than L3 and L4 for the other femoral nerves.

Fig 23 Anatomy of the femoral nerve

Motor units

A motor unit is the number of muscle fibres controlled by a single motor nerve fibre (an axon).

Very fine control requires very small motor units. In the middle ear the stapedius and tensor tympani muscles control the very delicate mechanism required for the transfer of sound waves into the inner ear. We call it hearing. Their motor units are between 2 and 3 muscle fibres per nerve axon*.

For the muscles controlling the eye, the motor units are about 4 to 8 muscle fibres supplied by a single nerve axon.*

In the course power muscles, such as the gluteus maximus, which is the buttock muscle and extends the hip, it is estimated that the motor units are between 1,500 and 2,000 muscle fibres controlled by a single motor axon.*

Somewhere it is written that the motor unit value of the quadricep muscles is about 450.*

These high numbers may be true for the majority of these power muscles, but it is not true for the distal area of the vastus medialis muscle, which by virtue of its nerve supply is defined by many as the vastus medialis oblique.

Cutting across a nerve bundle, one sees both motor and sensory axons wrapped in their protective Schwann cells. These have a lot of lipids and look white, and they act like electrical insulation. The axon is the dark bit in the middle. Motor and sensory axons look identical. Thus it would be too simplistic to suggest that all the axons seen in the large nerve to VMO are all motor nerves. Some, many possibly, are sensory but they must all have important function for nature to have evolved them, the sensory nerves for reflex Golgi tendon apparatus stretch receptors, for example.

An axon is the main connecting or conducting fibre of a nerve cell; other connecting fibres are called dendrites. All arise from and are supported by a cell body. The whole comprises the nerve cell.

In the sensory peripheral nerves, the cell body is lodged just outside the spinal canal in the dorsal root ganglion, and a dendrite passes into the spinal cord dorsal root to synapse with other cells in the substantia nigra and gelatinosa (as discussed later in 'How Pain Seems to Work'). The motor cell bodies, in contrast, are in the ventral root in the spinal column, and their axons exit via the ventral root. These roots join to form the peripheral nerves carrying both motor and sensory messages in their axons to and from the periphery. A sensory axon from a man's big toe may be 4 or even 5 ft long (up to 1.5 m). Elsewhere, like the brain, they may be very short from one cell to the next.

*These figures vary depending upon which author you read.

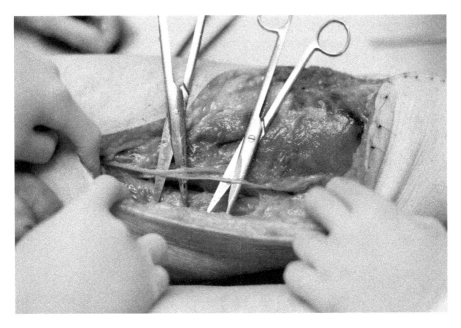

Fig 24 The large nerve to the VMO entering the muscle belly

Nerve to vastus medialis oblique

The nerve to the VMO part of the muscle is huge; for example, it is much bigger than the median nerve that supplies all the delicate functions of one half of the hand or the ulna nerve that supplies the other half of the hand. Big nerves with very many nerve fibres must have function. Nature did not evolve them to look pretty.

Fig 25 is the low power cross-section at this point, the left-hand end of the nerve in Fig 24. Fig 26 is showing one bundle in higher power to display the number of axons in each bundle.

Actually, nature only evolved a monster nerve to the distal vastus medialis in humans, with our bipedal gait and rather oddly designed knees that can permit both extension, flexion with roll back, and also rotation, all at the same time. Even the apes do not have a vastus medialis oblique.

Compare the bundle size of the nerve to the VMO to the leash of nerves passing under the inguinal ligament that supply all the other thigh muscles (see in Fig 27, page 70). There are fewer axons in the cross sections shown in Figs 28 and 29 (pages 71 and 72).

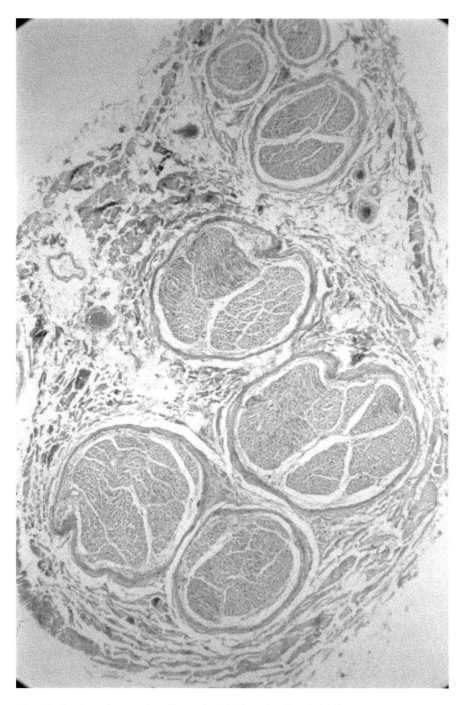

Fig 25 Section of nerve bundle to the VMO at the distal thigh, low power

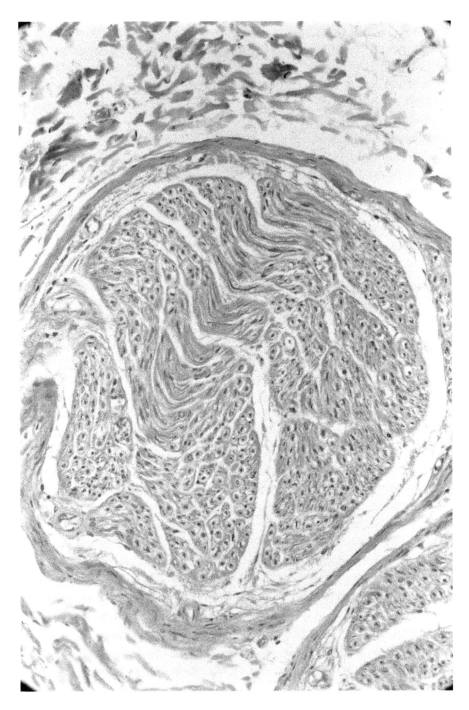

Fig 26 Nerve bundle to the VMO as it enters muscle; one bundle from Fig 25 at high power

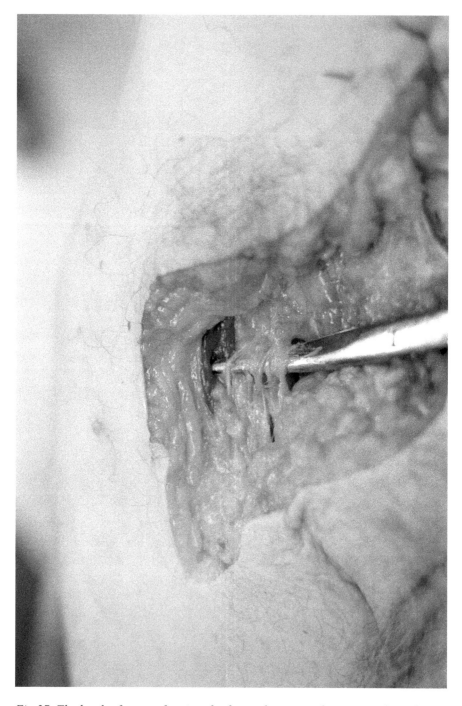

Fig 27 The leash of nerves forming the femoral nerve in the groin without the nerve to the VMO

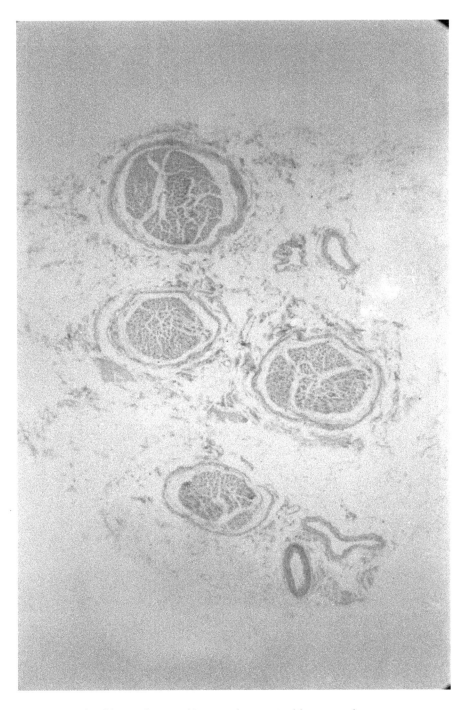

Fig 28 Leash of femoral nerve fibres at the inguinal ligament, low power

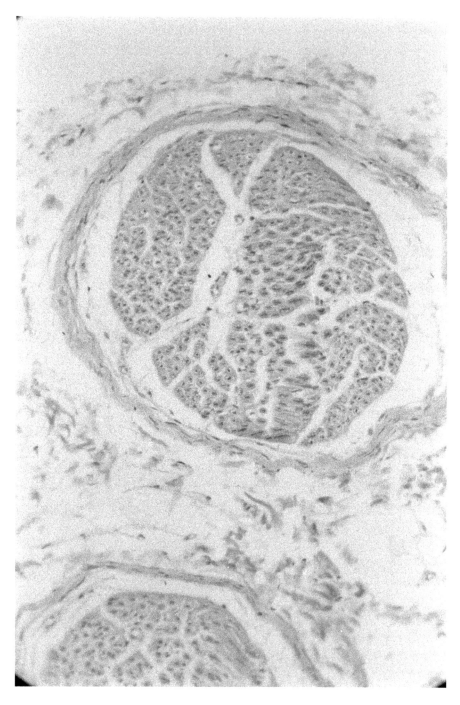

Fig 29 One of the nerves from the leash to the powerhouse muscles at the inguinal ligament from Fig 28, high power

The nerve to the VMO I have dissected out in a number of specimens from the inguinal ligament down. The anatomy is a thick nerve with no branches until it plunges into the VMO muscle.

Sometime the nerves to the vastus medialis and the rectus femoris seem intimate with it, but these bundles can be very simply separated from the big VMO nerve.

I have not pursued the nerve proximally (upwards) behind the abdominal cavity, but it is written somewhere that the fibres of the small branches to the vastus lateralis, vastus intermedius, rectus femoris, sartorius and vastus medialis arise from spinal levels L3, L4 and L5, and the much bigger nerve to the VMO arises from the upper lumbar levels, L1 and L2.

The nerves are formed of groups of axons wrapped in Schwann cells and further wrapped into bundles, and then the bundles into whole nerves by epineurium and perineurium. The Schwann cells are filled with lipids and look white and form both electrical insulation and also protection for the axon, or nerve fibre. The diameter of axons is related to their function: 20μ are fast axons both motor and sensory, and smaller $12\ \mu$ to $8\ \mu$ are to do with proprioception, pain, light touch, temperature and reflexes.[14]

Simply by looking at a cross-section of a nerve—any nerve—with a microscope, one cannot tell whether they are motor or sensory in function. Their size implies speed of conduction of their messages, and to some extent one can extrapolate their function[15].

The enormous number of fibres disappearing into the belly of the VMO must have function (all the bundles over the scissors in Fig 24, page 67 are the one nerve to the VMO). With a good hand lens, it is not possible to follow bundles of nerves through the belly of the muscle to the underlying joint capsule. They just disperse into the muscle. The implication is that the motor units of the VMO are small. I would hazard a guess at around 20, and possibly even less—and it is only a guess. That function must be to do with the delicacy of the control of the muscle.

---

[14] A 'μ' pronounced 'miu' is 0.001 mm (a millionth of a metre) or 0.000039 inch.

[15] Nerve fibres are all very small in diameter; by comparison, a red blood cell is about $8\ \mu$ diameter, and you can get about 4 million of those onto the head of a pin! A pain sensory axon from my big toe is about 1.2 m long. The nerve cell is just outside the spinal canal in the dorsal root ganglion and a dendrite continues into the dorsal root to synapse in the substantia gelatinosa.

That work I did at McGill, Montreal, in 1979,[16] but am ashamed to say I never really completed it to the point of publication. Basically, I dissected out the nerves to the quadriceps in a number of fresh cadavers. These photos of cross-sections of the nerves and the photo showing how the nerve branches and disappears into the belly of the muscle are all from one individual, a 56-year-old male who died of a heart attack. In this case, I weighed the various muscles and tried to compare the number of fibres in the cross-section slides to the muscles' weights. His VMO weighed about 450 gm. The other quadriceps muscles individually all weighed more. Even if only 50% of the fibres were motor, the implied motor unit value would be more than 10 times lower than in the other quadricep muscles, and one would then have to ask the question: 'Why so many sensory fibres? They too must all have some vital function.' There are also stretch and reflex controlling fibres exiting from the muscle belly and travelling in the nerve alongside the motor fibres. All are seen on the cross section with no obvious delineation.

(As a technical and sociological note, it is not so simple to get permissions to dissect fresh cadaver thighs. Families are not always that happy. I have not tried to repeat this study.)

In summary

I contend that the size of this nerve is very important. I believe it is a reflection of the motor unit value of the vastus medialis oblique muscle in comparison to motor unit values of the rest of the quadricep muscles, and this relates directly to its fine control function of steering. Steering is required, such that the patella, as it moves against the femoral groove, maintains the correct tension in the capsule, the retinacula and ligament structures of the knee and the correct pressures between the patellar articular facets and the femoral condyles for the hyaline cartilage to remain well nourished and healthy.

The muscle is big because it has a lot of work to do. Here there is a very much larger number of nerve fibres supplying a rather smaller muscle bulk. I believe that the motor units of this part of the muscle are very much smaller than in the rest of the quadriceps. Small motor units imply fine control and, one must add, an increased susceptibility to the inhibitory effects of pain.

The Vastus Medialis Oblique is a steering muscle. It is not a powerhouse muscle.

---

[16] There is a plethora of papers written if one looks up 'nerve to vastus medialis' on the web. The authors are all a little tenuous in drawing firm conclusions from their findings. They struggle to agree on the idea of the VMO and seem to back away from considering the motor unit values of this bit of muscle and the implication.

Nature needs a steering muscle

I would further my argument thus. The power muscles arise from the proximal (top end) of the femur, front lateral and posterior surfaces and the linea aspera at the back of the femoral shaft. Their muscle bundles combine to form the quadricep tendon that envelops the patella (the patella is technically a sesamoid bone). Their combined pull is both proximal and outwards on the patella. The patellar tendon attaches to the tibial tubercle, which creates an angle over the knee in the pulley system. This is the 'Q' Angle.

Observation of just how the knee moves—not just flexing and extending, but accommodating the rotation of the femur on the tibia from the movements of the hip, the subtalar joints in the ankle and the active rotation in directional changes in turning when walking, running and cutting, as in the 'Dummy Pass'—shows that there is great variation in the 'Q' Angle. The squeezing force generated by the bulk of the quadriceps, on the undersurfaces of the patella, and the underlying femoral condyles must be changed as the 'Q' Angle changes. That pressurisation of the joint surfaces is a function of the force created by the powerhouse muscles and the direction of application to the patellofemoral joint. The body weight does not change, but the inward corrective forces to counter the bowstring effect must change continuously to maintain the pressures in the physiological range in the patellofemoral joint according to the need. The VMO is positioned to apply that medialisation pull counteracting the bowstring effect of the angle in the pulley system; hence, the concept of the steering muscle and the powerhouse muscles (see Fig 5, page 19).

Description of the Femoral Nerve

The femoral nerve enters the thigh under the inguinal ligament in the groin just lateral to the midpoint. The vein is medial, the artery is in the middle and the nerve is lateral. The root values for the femoral nerve are L1, L2, L3, and L4 in most individuals. The muscles supplied are those of the front of the thigh—the four quadriceps, sartorius, rectus femoris and gracilis— and poor little articularis genu that pulls the synovial suprapatellar pouch up out of the patella's way.

VAN (Vein Artery Nerve) for anyone trying to remember this. Important if sticking needles into the artery and particularly if taking blood from

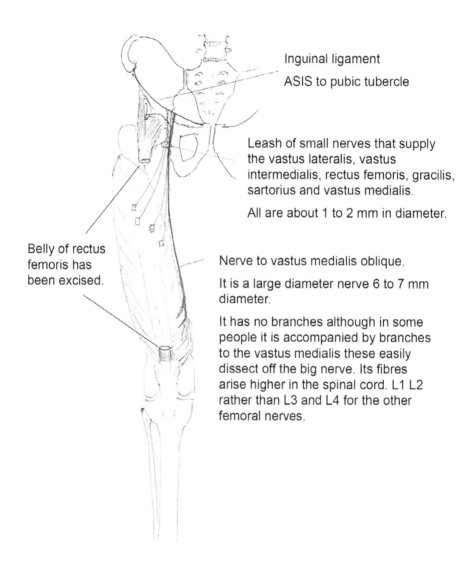

Inguinal ligament

ASIS to pubic tubercle

Leash of small nerves that supply the vastus lateralis, vastus intermedialis, rectus femoris, gracilis, sartorius and vastus medialis.

All are about 1 to 2 mm in diameter.

Belly of rectus femoris has been excised.

Nerve to vastus medialis oblique.

It is a large diameter nerve 6 to 7 mm diameter.

It has no branches although in some people it is accompanied by branches to the vastus medialis these easily dissect off the big nerve. Its fibres arise higher in the spinal cord. L1 L2 rather than L3 and L4 for the other femoral nerves.

Fig 30 Anatomy of the femoral nerve

babies. The hip lies right under the artery. Hip infections destroy the femoral head, Tom Smith's disease, a real risk from poor technique in taking blood from infants.

Normally, at the level of the inguinal ligament the nerve has broken up into a number of branches. All of these are quite small in their cross-sectional area, a couple of millimetres at the most, with the exception of the nerve to the vastus medialis oblique (the VMO). This is four or five times the cross-sectional area of even the largest of the other branches. With careful dissection, each of these branches can be dissected out and traced into the muscle it supplies.

Sometimes the nerve fibres to the midpart of the vastus medialis, rather than being a separate nerve bundle, are very intimate with the much bigger nerve to the VMO, but they can always be teased off from the larger nerve. The big nerve does not have any branches until it plunges into the belly of the muscle. This larger nerve, to the VMO, I described above.

One tends to focus on the powerhouse and steering muscles and their nerves. But there are other nerve functions. These nerves too are some of those in the leash that passes under the inguinal ligament and are also small (i.e. not all the visible axons are motor).

Other functions of the thigh muscles, and the mechanism to stop 'wobble'

Uneven wobble of the mass of the powerhouse muscles would alter the direction of the application of power to the patella and would distress the patellofemoral joint surfaces; indeed it does! Nature, in my opinion, has evolved two solutions to stop the wobble: the fascia lata and the sartorius, both of whose contractions appear to stabilise the bulk of the thigh muscles.

Fascia lata

The function of the fascia lata—the thickened band like a flattened tendon on the lateral side in the fascia that wraps the thigh muscles—in my view, is primarily to stop too much side-to-side wobble of the quadricep muscle mass as it applies its force to the top of the patella. It is tensioned by the tensor fascia latae muscle that arises on the outer edge of the front of the iliac crest. The fascia lata is inserted onto Gerdy's tubercle on the outer side of the front of the tibia. It benefits from the Starling Law effect of muscle contraction; that is, a muscle, if it is being stretched, can generate more force. The fascia lata is lengthened with knee flexion, which might generate a Starling effect to prepare for the act of extension by the quads. The quads action to extend the knee could cause wobble in the line of pull, and wobble would be bad news for the patellofemoral joint surfaces.

Sartorius

This muscle runs across the front of the thigh and inserts onto the medial upper tibia. It too could benefit from a Starling Law effect as above. Its role seems to me to be part of the stabilisation of the quadricep bulk as they work.

Chapter 12

Articular Surfaces

Hyaline cartilage

Chondromalacia patellae

Joints need to move; this is an absolute for healthy diarthrodial joints. A diarthrodial joint is one hyaline cartilage surface moving on another. The cartilage behaves like a firm sponge. Squeezed by movement the fluid in the matrix is squeezed out, release the pressure and the joint or synovial fluid moves back into the cartilage matrix. Fluid being squeezed out and in by the pressure and movement is the only source of nourishment of the chondrocytes in the matrix of the cartilage (see Fig 31, page 80).

Nutrition of hyaline cartilage

Movement actually seems to make the synovium more comfortable. Patients on CPM (continuous passive movement) machines post-op rarely need analgesia (painkillers).

The articular-bearing surfaces of any joint that permits movement is hyaline cartilage. This is the shiny stuff on the joint surfaces that one can see in any butcher's shop. The word 'cartilage' is not to be confused with the menisci of the knee, often called 'cartilages', as in: 'I have had my cartilage removed.' The limb joints are all diarthrodial joints. The anatomy of this hyaline cartilage is well described. The functional significance of its physiology seems not so well appreciated.

In simple terms, there is an arrangement of collagen fibres apparently produced by chondrocytes that arch up from the underlying, or subchondral, bone to curve over just below the joint surface and descend back to the bone. Between these arcading fibres are the chondrocytes, the cartilage cells. In between the chondrocytes and the collagen fibres is a solution that is primarily proteoglycans (PG) molecules, glycosaminoglycans (GAG) molecules, hyaluronic acid molecules with 'link protein' attaching the GAGs—forming structures like long hairy caterpillars at a molecular level—plus the mineral molecules that make up body fluids; and all suspended in what is, in effect, synovial fluid.

NB The thickness of the hyaline cartilage, thinned when under load

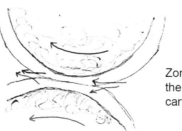

Zone of increasing pressure, fluid being squeezed out of the matrix

Zone of pressure reducing, the joint fluid re-enters the cartilage matrix

Fig 31 How fluid is squeezed out as pressure is applied to hyaline cartilage and how it goes back in as pressure is relieved

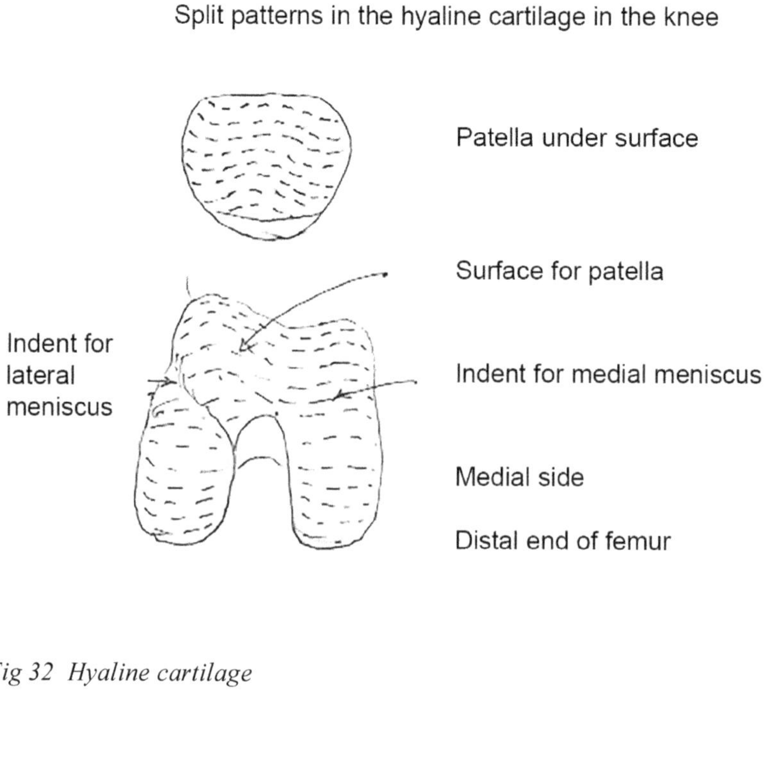

Split patterns in the hyaline cartilage in the knee

Patella under surface

Surface for patella

Indent for lateral meniscus

Indent for medial meniscus

Medial side

Distal end of femur

Fig 32 Hyaline cartilage

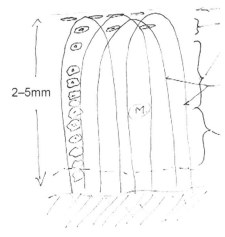

Surface zone of flat cells

Zone of oval cells

Zone of round cells becoming columnar

Collagen fibres, rising from the bone, arching at the surface and back to the bone

Zone of chondrocytes apparently without nucleii

Tidemark zone of calcification

Subchondral bone

2–5mm

Arcading collagen fibres

Chondrocytes; collagen fibres all suspended in what is essentially synovial joint fluid

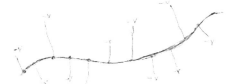

A complex molecule of PG and GAG molecules attached by link protein to a hyaluronic acid molecule.

These are the complex molecules dissolved in the fluid of the cartilage matrix.

In this case it would be from an adolescent as there are both chondroitin sulphate and keratin sulphate molecules.

NB All the sulphate molecules are negatively charged and repel each other.

Fig 33 The cartilage matrix

At and just under the joint surface, the cells are flatter and seem to be evenly spread. A little deeper and they take on a more oval form; this is still at the level where the collagen fibres are arching. Deeper still, where the fibres are parallel to each other and at right angles to the surface of the joint and the bone, the chondrocytes are in columns. The deepest cells just above the bone surface seem to be almost lifeless, as they possess no nuclei on staining. There is a line of calcification just above the bone, which may be an expression of low oxygen tension. Long term, chronic hypoxia is a potent cause for calcification in the body.

Cartilage is directional stuff. It was evolved to move in particular directions only. It is not tolerant of shear. In about 1948 a bored youth was learning his anatomy and rather angrily repeatedly stabbed the hyaline surface of the joint in front of him with his pen nib. He then noticed that the dots of ink formed splits. When he stabbed the surfaces of other joints, the patterns of the splits were always in the same directions. He eventually did the same for most of the joints of the body, and the split directions were always consistent. In other words, he demonstrated that cartilage is directional stuff. The alignment of the collagen fibres was directional and not haphazard, although at that time microscopy was not able to define this (see Fig 32, page 80). This was long before the introduction of the electron microscope and the understanding of the anatomy of hyaline cartilage.

The hyaluronic acid molecule is a long chain. At intervals along the chain, attached by link protein, there are GAG molecules, keratan sulphate and chondroitin sulphate. The free ends of these GAG molecules are electrically charged. The charges are all negative and so mutually repulse. The result is that the ends of these molecules are repelled from each other (see Fig 33, page 81).

As stated above, when cartilage is under load it behaves like a firm sponge; some of the fluid is squeezed out of the matrix as pressure is applied during movement. When the pressure on the surface is relieved, the molecules try to move apart and the matrix can expand again, drawing fluid back into the matrix.

This circulation of joint fluid through the matrix is the ONLY source of nourishment and respiration for the chondrocytes (see Fig 31, page 80).

One consequence of this is that the metabolic rate of chondrocytes is very slow; it may even be anoxic (i.e. not needing oxygen). Chondrocytes do metabolise and are responsible for the production of the matrix collagen and the chemicals, PGs and GAGs. It is extremely rare to see cell division on microscopic examination of adult hyaline cartilage. So much so, that if one does see mitochondria and a mitosis—that is, the splitting of cells as they grow—on histological examination, it was taught that this should be considered to be a chondrosarcoma, a rare cancer of the chondrocytes, until proved otherwise.

While caution is appreciated, these cells do sometimes have to do their job. One obvious job is to grow the articular surfaces from tiny, as in a child, through the adolescent growth spurt to adulthood. Chondroitin sulphate is a long chain molecule and produces softer cartilage than keratin sulphate. Chondroitin sulphate is found in children and adolescents. Keratin sulphate is only found in adults. The softer cartilage of youth is more easily squeezed and distorted and better irrigated by synovial fluid, and hence better chondrocyte nourishment than in the adult.

Another consequence is that it has been written—derivative facts—and is widely believed, that hyaline cartilage cannot heal. I disagree with this statement, and more modern academic studies now agree that there does seem to be an ability of chondrocytes to 'wake up' and initiate a degree of repair. A simple example is the fracture of the medial malleolus in the ankle, which is through the hyaline cartilage. It repairs, without consequence if properly realigned! Loose bodies are covered in hyaline cartilage, as are osteophytes, which form at the edges of articular surfaces in osteoarthritis. Hyaline cartilage can heal.

The pressures in adult, diarthrodial joints in different animal species have been determined. It would seem that they all function in a very similar pressure per unit area range right across the adult animal spectrum: 25 to 33 dynes/mm (old paper; old units).

The implications of the above are:

1. If there is insufficient pressure, there is not enough deformation to promote a movement of synovial fluid into and out from the matrix, reducing the nourishment of the chondrocytes and their ability to maintain the matrix.
2. Too much pressure between the joint surfaces and shear forces in directions for which the cartilage is not aligned, and mechanical crushing, will result in damage. Deep splits in the matrix have been demonstrated (circa 1980).
3. For good cartilage health there needs to be the correct directional movement in the correct pressure range. Anything else will result in unhealthy cartilage or damage.

Either way—shear, undernourished or overpressurised—there will be a potential for the release of the chemicals that make up the matrix (PG and

GAG) and collagen products, and the synovium will have to work harder to clear up the detritus.

(I had two patients who had walked around for some months with locked knees. On arthroscopy there were big bucket-handle tears of the medial menisci still lying displaced through the intercondylar notch. After removal of the torn meniscus in each case, examination of the hyaline cartilage on the femoral condyles that had been subjected to constant abnormal pressure showed that a piece of the hyaline cartilage was loose and almost detached. I removed them both, exposing subchondral bone; ulcers about 10 mm x 7.5 mm in each case.

They were encouraged to fully weight-bear straight away and return to normal function as quickly as possible. Recovery was uneventful. After six months I confess that I was curious, and so about eight or nine months post original arthroscopy I 'scoped' them again. To my surprise, there was no hyaline cartilage ulceration. The areas were filled in completely with something that looked like hyaline cartilage. I did not take samples, but to my eye they had healed.)

Synovium

The lining membrane of a joint is called synovium. One function of synovium is to produce synovial fluid; the other function is to clean up any debris by a phagocytic action, where the synovial cells envelop the debris molecules and bits. An excess of PG and GAG release will overstimulate the synovium. If overworked, it will become a bit inflamed. It looks pink and develops fingerlike fimbria. On arthroscopy it can look like fronds of seaweed. The synovial cells, which produce the joint fluid, will also overproduce, and hence the effusion (fluid in the joint). In a full-blown arthritis or inflammation of the joint, the overworked lytic mechanisms will leak lytic enzymes into the joint fluid and bathe all the articular surfaces, softening them and predisposing them to mechanical damage.

I have stated that synovium is very sensitive to pain, much more so when inflamed. Clinically, this is recognised as a warm, sensitive, swollen, active arthritis, as opposed to the same joint when it is calmed down with medication, when it would be described as a joint showing arthrosis (i.e. signs of damage but not hot and angry or inflamed!).

In a joint like the knee, with inflammation the enzyme-rich fluid produced in one area is also bathing the healthy cartilage elsewhere and possibly softening it, predisposing to damage elsewhere. What was noticed in the 1980s—when we extended our indications for medial unicompartmental joint replacement, where we were pushing the boundaries a little because we ignored some early arthritic changes in the lateral compartments—was that after putting an artificial joint in medially, the lateral compartments became healthy again. This also occurred when we did patelloplasties (operations to reshape the undersurfaces of the patellae). This is not practised by many orthopaedic surgeons (more's the pity).

Synovial fluid is not the most nutritious of body fluids. Chondrocyte cells have a tough time to survive, hence their slow metabolic rate. As stated above, chondroitin sulphate is a longer chain than keratin sulphate. It produces a softer, more elastic cartilage than keratin sulphate. Chondroitin sulphate is the chemical found in the hyaline cartilage in children and adolescents. In adults it is almost exclusively keratin sulphate that is present. In one's late teens and early 20s it is a changing mixture. One sees individuals in late teens with adult weight and muscle bulk but still with rather delicate joints. All one can advise is for them to keep fit and get older!

Joints and their articular surfaces obviously must grow in size during youth. There must be reproduction of chondrocyte cells. They must be capable of making more hyaline cartilage to cover the growing bone ends. Their metabolism would appear to be a little faster than in adulthood, which implies that the nutrition of the cells must be better. The chondroitin hyaline cartilage is softer and deforms more easily under the lesser loads in children's joints. It may be more susceptible to shear forces damaging it. It permits a faster movement of synovial fluid through the matrix of the cartilage surfaces that would support a faster metabolism in the chondrocytes.

Adults need to be more resilient to the hard knocks of life and the greater pressures of their heavier weight. Keratin sulphate makes for a stiffer matrix.

There is, however, evidence that hyaline cartilage can be generated in adulthood. In osteoarthritis (the wear and tear arthritis of ageing) there is all too often the development of osteophytes. These are new bone excrescences that develop along the edges of the areas of wear on the articular surface. They have hyaline cartilage on their surfaces. Where does it come from? Chondrocytes must be able to produce it.

These are points in favour of the argument that hyaline cartilage has reparative potential. Providing that the ideal conditions for its nutrition, movement in the right direction and correct loading are there, healing will occur.

If the mechanical axis of the loading through the joint is disturbed by malalignment—many reasons for this are possible—and the cartilage is not working in its optimum pressure range and direction and is subject to abnormal shear movements, it may well break down and not repair, and will be further damaged.

There are surgical procedures that have endeavoured to implant hyaline cartilage onto eburnated bone of femoral condyles. Initially, they did not report very encouraging results. If the surgeon had not also addressed the overloading and shear, I am not surprised.

Fibrocartilage

This needs to be discussed. It is also an attempt to repair an articular surface ulcer, but it looks greyish with an arthroscope. There is a procedure of drilling eburnated bone (cartilage completely worn off to expose subchondral bone). It rejoiced in the name of the Priddy procedure. Combined with early resumption of movement, with CPM for example, it can result in functioning surfaces, albeit probably fibrocartilage.

Causes of arthritis

Also note that the cause of the arthritic process may be very different: gout, pseudo gout, rheumatoid, and wear and tear, associated with various infections and diseases. There are about 60 different causes for acute arthritis and about half that for chronic arthritis, but in all, the end result is a similar process of swollen overactive synovium. All will be painful and all, therefore, will inhibit steering muscle function.

(As a clinical sign, a little fluid in a joint, even if it is not very symptomatic, suggests that at least part of the interior of that joint is not entirely 'happy'. By contrast, a completely dry joint, even in the presence of a litany of dramatic complaints, testifies that things are pretty healthy inside the joint.)

Chapter 13

The Patella

The kneecap, or patella, is classified as a sesamoid bone. It is the largest sesamoid in the body. A sesamoid is a bone that is within a tendon, usually where the tendon slides over a bony prominence. It is a way that nature protects the tendon and the underlying articular surface. When a tendon is loaded over a prominence, the tendon distorts and reduces its internal blood supply by a 'wringing' out of the tissues. The bone does not distort. A sesamoid bone may also act as a fulcrum, improving the leverage so that the force generated by the muscle is more efficiently used. This certainly seems to be the case in the knee.

The patella has articular (hyaline) cartilage on the surfaces that transfer the pressure load. These surfaces are called facets. These patellar facets articulate with the front of the femoral condyles and the sides of the intercondylar notch, also covered in articular cartilage. As the femoral condyles are separated by the intercondylar notch, each facet articulates with a specific area.

During movement, there is the sliding effect and also a rolling effect of the patella, such that the loaded area moves distally and onto both side facets as the knee bends, as demonstrated by Dr David Burke, MD. This action evidently helps with cartilage nutrition.

The thickness of the patella helps mechanically, serving to improve leverage. It is of interest that after the operation of patellectomy (i.e. removal of the bone that is done occasionally for severe fractures) the tendon, once it has healed, eventually thickens up to about the same thickness as that of the patella. This process, in my experience, seems to take up to three years, or possibly a little longer.

The rolling effect demonstrates well the mechanism required for nutrition of chondrocytes in hyaline cartilage, a mechanism that must occur in every joint for satisfactory cartilage nutrition and health. It is the squeezing out of fluid from the matrix—in which dwell the chondrocytes—when under load and the return of synovial joint fluid back into the matrix as the pressure is diminished that is the sole source of nutrition and possibly respiration of the chondrocytes. See diagram of cartilage nutrition (Fig 33, page 81).

Functions of the patella

- It is evidently a mechanism for transferring tension load.
- It improves the mechanical advantage of the quadricep tendon by virtue of its thickness.
- The patella protects the front of the femoral condyles from direct trauma.
- By its combined sliding action and its tilting, such that the loaded area moves up and down the undersurface of the patella, it ensures nourishment of the cartilage of the femoral condyle and the cartilage of the undersurface of the patella itself.
- **Most importantly, it ensures that the pull from the quadricep muscles on the tibial tubercle is always in the midline of the knee joint.**

But it does not follow that the pressures under the patella are in the optimal pressure range without good VMO function. Unequal loading of the facets in this function is the root cause for most of the problems with the patellofemoral joint.

When people started taking skyline patellar views of the bone, they could see the clear gap on X-ray films that represents two thicknesses of hyaline cartilage, one on each surface. (Hyaline cartilage is invisible to X-rays.) If the gaps were the same on both sides, the simple interpretation was that the joints were normal. If the bone was tilted and the gaps were different thicknesses, people became more interested. Actually, it is quite possible to have the two pairs of surfaces in contact with very different pressure loads, medial and lateral.

In the physics lab at school there were some very highly polished blocks of steel. These could be placed one directly on top of the other, and the presumption was that the pressure per unit area between the surfaces was the same all over. Slide the top block out to one side so that it overhangs the lower block, and just before it over balances, almost all the weight—and therefore the pressure—is concentrated along the edge of the lower block, even though the supporting surfaces appear to be in contact.

The same principle is seen in architecture. To create a roof, one could corbel out to cross the gap, and the contact pressure would be increased towards the edge of the stone blocks. These thoughts seemed to have been missed by some in orthopaedics evaluating shoot through or skyline patellofemoral X-ray films.

Lateral

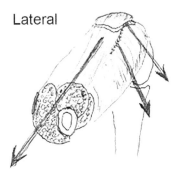

Medial

P   p

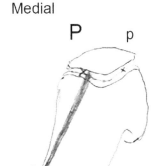

The effect of VMO
contraction on the
pressures under the
patella.

The power force is at 90°
on the lateral facet but
produces a shear force
under the medial side.

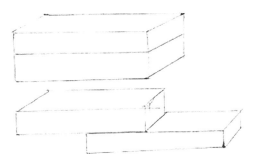

2 highly polished steel
blocks. The pressures are
equal all over the contact
surfaces.

Just prior to tipping the
pressure is concentrated at
the tipping point.

But the surfaces still **appear** to be together. This interpretation was not
appreciated when skyline patella views were being looked at.

Fig 34 Pressure in contact surfaces

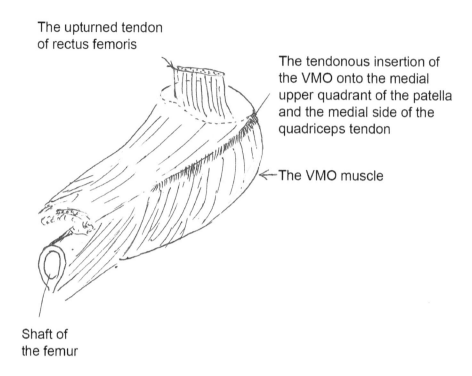

The upturned tendon
of rectus femoris

The tendonous insertion of
the VMO onto the medial
upper quadrant of the patella
and the medial side of the
quadriceps tendon

←The VMO muscle

Shaft of
the femur

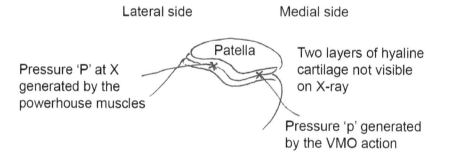

Lateral side

Medial side

Pressure 'P' at X
generated by the
powerhouse muscles

Patella

Two layers of hyaline
cartilage not visible
on X-ray

Pressure 'p' generated
by the VMO action

NB The powerhouse pull is at 90° to the facets in the lateral
contact area but produces an oblique shear force in the medial
side of the patello femoral joint. The VMO pulls the force to
90° across the contact area.

Fig 35 Skyline diagram of the patellofemoral joint

Hunter's cap patella

This is an anomaly of the patella that is seen in late teens and adults. It is a little more common in females. The term is derived from the X-ray appearance of the patella when taken in the 'shoot through' manner, giving a cross-section. These days CT scans are used to give the same cross-sectional view. On a normal patellar the articular surfaces are smoothly curved, with a slight keel in the middle (like certain Chinese and Mongolian bows). Look at the pictures. The hunter's cap patella develops without a medial articular surface. Quite often they are unilateral (i.e. in one leg only). I believe that they are all secondary to a failure of the VMO muscle to apply enough pulling force during development. Many patients will give a history of some sort of injury in early life often forgotten about. In some circles hunter's cap patellae seem to create lots of excitement (see Fig 36 below).

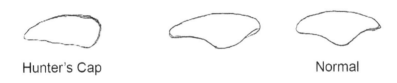

Hunter's Cap   Normal

Types of patella seen in 'normal' knees

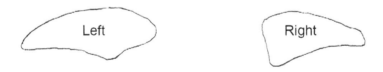

Tracing of the patellae of a man, aged 47.
At the age of ten he had suffered an accident that injured his thigh and inside of his knee. He recalls that it took a very long time to heal. He has always had a weak and painful right leg.

Fig 36 Hunter's cap patellae

'Skyline' patella views

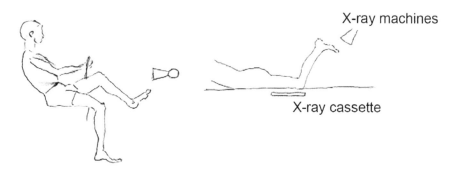

Fig 37 Position for getting a skyline patellar view X-ray film

There were some studies years ago taking chicken bones from embryos or very young chicks and growing them on tissue cultures. When they had grown, they were compared to bones left to grow in the creature. In effect, one bone grew with muscles attached and the other grew with no muscles attached. Both grew to the same length and size, but the one with no muscle attachments did not develop any of the lumps and bumps we now recognise as being produced by the muscles. In well-muscled human males these bone markings are much greater than in delicate females. No VMO function equals no medial forces and no development of the medial side of the patella.

I have seen the condition in a number of patients who have sustained quite major knee injury in their youth—for example, from RTAs (slang for road traffic accidents) or from being kicked by a horse—and often with prolonged healing times due to infection, which has resulted in poor or no medial condyle and sometimes chronic lateral subluxation (dislocation) of the patella. In their other leg the development of the patella was normal.

After years of poor use of the muscle, these patients require a bit of help to start to recognise their VMO muscle and be able to make it function. With a little patience and persistence doing the exercise, the reward can be normal function. The surgeon may have had to do something as well to get them going.

(One of my physiotherapists in the British Columbian bush used a TENS machine turned up as a muscle stimulator in reluctant VMOs. It worked very well.)

Much is made in the orthopaedic and related literature of the shapes of patellae and the contribution to patellofemoral pain and problems this causes. The shapes have been graded: I–IV or A–C. I believe that this concern is a little misplaced. I really do not believe that the shape need be a cause for persistent knee pain. This is not to say that it may not reflect the cause for anterior knee pain, but a patient with an anomalously shaped patella may be rendered entirely pain free, and without its excision!

The underdevelopment of the medial side of the patella is also seen in people, usually females, who have had persistent and unsuccessfully treated anterior knee problems during their adolescent growth spurt.

In one unusual case, a woman had endured a dislocating patella from the age of 14 to the age of 67, when I saw her for increasing knee pain. I noted that her patella was completely flat on the undersurface and there was no intercondylar notch on the femur. The lateral condyle of the femur was low. As the knee was bent beyond 5 degrees, the patella slipped laterally onto the side of the lateral femoral condyle. Her other knee was quite normal.

(The solution I chose was to turn the patella over and reshape it, carve an intercondylar notch on the femur, perform a lateral release of the knee capsule and perform a combined anterior advancement and realignment (Elmslie-Trillat plus a Maquet) procedure of the patellar tendon, fixed with one screw. I think I also dissected up and advanced her vastus medialis oblique muscle, such as it was. That, plus immediate passive movement (CPM) and specific re-education of the medialising elements of her quadriceps, completely restored normal and pain-free function over a period of about six months.)

I have been surprised as to why orthopaedic surgeons have failed to tackle patellofemoral problems, except that it does require a full understanding of the mechanisms of control of the patellofemoral joint and the courage of one's convictions to perform procedures not wholly sanctioned by the majority. A combination of elevation of the tibial tubercle, realignment of the tibial tubercle and the patellar tendon, reshaping the patella, patelloplasty and reattaching or advancing the vastus medialis oblique muscle itself will cure it. Reawakening of the VMO is needed post-op. It may sound a lot, but surgery that does not address all the elements of a problem often results in suboptimal results. It does not take very long, but 'get it right', and the patients are very grateful. One does sometimes have to overcome the effects of previous, failed treatments and persuade the patient to work at the exercises in the initial rehab phase. Sadly, and quite often, there is a strong, iatrogenic nihilism about the prospects of recovery.

As an aside, look at the skyline X-ray view I have drawn and then at the diagram of the steel blocks (see Figs 34 and 35, pages 89 and 90). The point is that although the surfaces appear to be in contact on the X-ray film, it does not mean that the pressures between the surfaces can be assumed to be equal. Now extend your thinking to the nutrition of chondrocytes and the physical conditions required for that.

There was a vogue for plastic patellar replacements. While I used them in some total knee replacements, I preferred the combination of elevation and medialisation of the tibial tubercle and VMO re-education. (See the Elmslie-Trillat and Maquet in the Appendix for simple patellofemoral arthritic problems.)

Patellectomy

This is the name of the operation that removes part or all of the patella. In the past it was done quite often. It is my belief that it does have a place, after trauma, but that in the past it was overused. I do not think it should have a place in the management of anterior knee pain. The clinician's role should be to identify which tissue appears to be responsible for the origin of the patient's pain, and then to deal with it.

Remember the example of the needle. Stab your knee with a needle. Observe the sensations that YOU experience: 'BL**DY OATH!' Yet if one were to try to locate the site of entry of the needle into the knee with an arthroscope, it really is not possible. The message is that the actual amount of tissue causing a patient to complain of crippling pain may not be very big. This is why so many people continue with 'chronic' pain for years.

I saw a number of people, all men, who presented to me with rather dull and non-specific knee pain, all of whom had had patellectomies for fractures. They all responded well to being taught how to get their VMOs working again.

I offer another, rather sad, case of a man over 60 who had worn shorts for 50 years because he could not tolerate the discomfort of trousers rubbing over his knees. This was in Canada, where it gets very cold. He was experiencing increasing knee pain and loss of movement. It was late in the year.

He had been injured as a child and he had been treated with bilateral patellectomy. There was neuroma-like hypersensitivity over one knee, in the scar, and the other knee had a fairly large bony remnant, which seemed to be causing pain. The patellar tendons on both knees had hypertrophied to over 2cm thickness. He had no vastus medialis oblique function detectable.

Simple excision of the site of the neuroma-like pain was performed on one side and excision of the bony lump from within the quadricep tendon on the other. Also arthroscopic removal of some fimbria and synovial scars in both knees. Personal instruction in VMO control was by myself.

He returned at six weeks to my follow-up clinic pleased as punch, wearing long trousers for the first time in nearly 50 years and able to play in the snow, something denied to him almost all his life. He now displayed active VMO function!

Patellar anomalies

Bipartite patella, and very occasionally tripartite, occurs; and because both can be a bit lumpy, they can cause patellar tracking problems and pain. The solution is simply to excise the extra bit of the patella, taking care not to set off bleeding from the anastomosing blood vessels around the patella, which one of my less skilled juniors did!

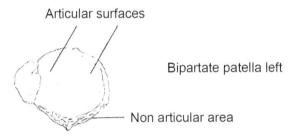

Fig 38 Bipartite patella

Chapter 14

How Pain Seems to Work

I have stated the premise that pain causes incoordination. It also causes wasting of muscles. Muscle-wasting will occur with lack of use, but it seems to occur surprisingly rapidly in the presence of localised pain. I have measured up to 1 inch (2.5 cm) of wasting in the quadriceps of athletes after open medial arthrotomies (an incision into a joint is an arthrotomy—sorry, a technical term) in the first 36 to 48 hours after the surgery. Incision into the medial side of the knee is very much more painful than the lateral side, as I can testify. Understanding how pain seems to work in orthopaedic patients helps in managing their problems. Pain seems to produce more wasting than can be explained simply by disuse.[17]

This section is a gross simplification of what happens, I admit, but it seems to work, in that local anaesthetic injected into a bit of tissue triggering pain can render an almost hysterical individual into one behaving normally and rationally. As the local wears off, they return to their bizarre

---

[17] This principle applies to all joints. As an illustration of this pain inhibition causing wasting, I recall a motorcycle-riding, bodybuilder who came off onto his right, dominant shoulder. There was a fracture of the neck of his glenoid, severe skin abrasions and a lot of bruising. Time is a great healer, and with progressive pendular exercises and the gentle administrations of his dear wife he appeared to be fully recovered, except that his infraspinatus muscle, on the scapula, just refused to reappear and his life as a competitive bodybuilder was destroyed.

One should not smile, but for him it was very important, even though he was back at work. I considered damage to the small branch of the suprascapular nerve, which winds around the outer end of the scapular spine to supply this muscle. I phoned a famous colleague, Dr Melzack, famous for his gate control theory of pain. He was able to do a very sophisticated electromyelogram study but could find no evidence of nerve damage. A further clinical examination, and the patient's report that he usually slept on his front on their rather firm-surfaced mattress, revealed a small but very tender site in the posterior rotator cuff, trapped, I contend, when his arm was in the fully abducted position needed to lie on his front.

My management of this sort of rotator cuff pinching problem was advice to sleep on a softer surface (do not confuse texture of the surface of a bed with the shape of a bed), to use a non-steroidal anti-inflammatory in the mornings for a couple of weeks, and often a very small localised injection of an anti-inflammatory steroid like triamcinolone (never use Depo-Medrone, please) and sometimes to change sides of the bed with one's partner so that you find a different position in which to sleep.

I injected a small quantity of steroid diluted in local anaesthetic solution into the painful site, plus, of course, all the good advice. Six weeks later, this after months of rehab and gym work, joy of joys, his infraspinatus was fully restored. Pain inhibition had caused the muscle-wasting!

presentations. Cure the pain permanently, and they remain normal. In the chronic knee pain population this bizarre behaviour only really applies to the scar neuroma type of pains and some capsular damage, but locating and removing the source of such a patient's pain is still the imperative of the medical personnel. In the acute situations, achieving some movement is surprisingly helpful in reducing what can be excruciating pain. CPM (continuous passive movement) is one such modality.

Do not deny the patient their pain, however bizarre or exaggerated their presentation seems. So often in the past, after outpatient visits and a string of negative clinical findings and investigations, there has been a tendency to say to the patient that 'nothing orthopaedic can be found'. The implication is that there is nothing there or that it is all in their head. This is particularly true when compensation is being claimed. Understandably, the patient may be quite upset.

(These thoughts were part of my teaching concerning back pain and whiplash patients but are occasionally very applicable to knee problems, particularly in the presence of previous trauma.)

In fact, for these poor people it is all in their head! If the brain's cortex is receiving pain messages, the individual will express that they are feeling pain. The question is therefore, where are all these pain messages in patients being generated?

There are very real effects of a psychosocial nature in the expression of pain. The same stimulus of pain receptors on the rugby pitch or in a bar on a Saturday night will not produce the same complaints as those produced in a car accident, after the game or in an accident at work, particularly when large sums of money might hang on the expression of symptoms. I do not propose to discuss this here beyond pointing out that the pain receptors out in the periphery are sending out the same messages in all cases. It is how the messages are processed and perceived on the brain's cortex that gives the patient their symptoms.

Exquisite pain may be produced by the triggering of a very small piece of tissue. This we have demonstrated by sticking a needle into one's fingertip, or deep into a knee! There can be less-than-obvious structures in and around the knee that can cause most distressing pain: a neuroma in a scar; a 'trigger point', whatever that might be; tissue scarring; tendonitis; anything synovial, such as a plica or even inflammatory synovial fimbria.

The simplest route to the diagnosis of this sort of pain is to gently palpate the part to localise the site of the pain. (Neuroma pain is electric, exquisite and very localised. One can touch it once and then the patient refuses further contact!) Then, clinician, think of the parts involved: that is, the anatomic structures of that site. Sometimes it is of value to then infiltrate with small volumes of local anaesthetic. Thus, such sites can readily be identified. The inclusion of a little anti-inflammatory steroid with the local anaesthetic can often achieve 'miracle' cures, although rarely permanent in the case of neuromas, in my experience.

(Please, do not infiltrate with Depo-Medrone, nor accept it. Only use Depo-Medrone if you want tissue atrophy. It is an obsolete drug for most soft-tissue problems.) Also, please, Marcaine causes three or four seconds of burning pain. Mix it with lignocaine (Lidocaine), which is almost immediate in its effect, to be kind to your patient.

Neuroma

A neuroma is a little whorl of axons, the actual nerve fibres, that can occur when a nerve has been cut and starts to heal. The healing axons that cannot find their way into the distal end of the sheath of Schwann cells form a little ball. Neuromas can be microscopically small. Normally, the Schwann cells wrap around the axons and both protect and electrically insulate them.

My message is that a very small bit of damaged tissue sending out pain messages may cause disabling symptomatology and muscle atrophy. How might this be?

Practical advice for doctors
Treatment of this sort of neuroma pain is simple, once you have thought about it; it is excision, often under local anaesthetic, of the actual piece of tissue with the neuroma in it. Sending the piece to histology is not worth it, as the neuroma is very small and is often missed in cutting the histological sections. The test is, what does the patient feel? Interestingly, once a neuroma is excised, it does not reform. I do not know why.

For trigger-point pain, in a scar for instance, the addition of some anti-inflammatory steroid to the local anaesthetic agent injected with precision into the site of the pain can cure it. The local anaesthetic acts both to dilute the steroid and to indicate that the injection is into the exact site causing the pain. Sometimes very little more than a drop in exactly the right place can cure longstanding problems. (Whiplash neck pains and tennis elbow respond very well). (Mix about 5:1, local:steroid.)

In tendonitis a very small injecting using a 29-gauge needle (absolute minimum quantity because one does not want to weaken the tendon) can bring dramatic relief.

Short-acting local anaesthetics like lignocaine will give relief for two hours; Bupivacaine or Marcaine will give 10 to 12 hours of relief, but Marcaine burns painfully for a few seconds after injection. These local anaesthetics are often premixed with adrenalin, which causes the small blood vessels to contract and so limits bleeding. But adrenalin injected into the skin also stings greatly. This can also be mitigated by mixing with lignocaine.

Different steroids will start acting with different delays from injection: dexamethasone and betamethasone within 24 hours; triamcinolone acetomide, and Celestone in North America, also within about 24 to 36 hours. Depo-Medrone, by contrast, takes up to 10 days to start its effect. It will continue to cause tissue atrophy for months. It also leaves a deposit in the tissues. Please do not use Depo-Medrone if you do not want tissues to atrophy.

Clinician, remember also that one's needle has been in very painful tissue, and the pain may be temporarily worse as the local wears off. Explaining this to the patient, giving some simple analgesia—I use Motrin or Ibuprofen—can help. It may also have a placebo effect. Placebo effect has a demonstrable release of endorphin in the spinal column. It all helps the patient deal with their problem.

Substantia gelatinosa

This is an area in the spinal cord where nerves carrying pain messages synapse with other nerves to pass the message along.

The nociceptor, or pain receptor, is served by an axon from a sensory nerve cell whose cell body is in the dorsal root ganglion, just outside the bony spinal canal. (The axon is the 'wire' that carries the message.) An axon from a man's toe can be about 4–5 ft long, the distance from the toe to the middle of the back. The message passes up the axon into the posterior horn of the spinal cord, where there is a synapse. A synapse is the structure whereby the electrochemical message in one nerve cell is transferred to another nerve cell, or cells, chemically. The pain message is thus transported in another axon that crosses to the other side of the spinal cord and turns up the spinothalamic tract to the area of the hind/mid brain, the thalamus. There the pain message again passes a synapse to another axon and yet a further axon before it is experienced on the cortex as a pain sensation.

At each of these synapses there is the possibility that the message can be passed to other functions of the nervous system. There is a measurable speed of axon transmission—faster in the thicker fibres—and of the time it takes for a message to cross a synapse.

> One of the mysteries of the professional athlete–like a batsman in cricket–is just how he can move his bat in time to score a run off a fast ball, presuming that the neural message must start when the light hits the back of his eyeball and has to travel through the brain and be expressed out in the limb in fine-control movements. And all that without him falling over!

The substantia gelatinosa is the area in the posterior horn of the spinal column where these first synapses occur, between the pain message fibre and the ongoing message up the spinal cord to the brain.

A simple observation would suggest that there must be other effects of a pain message arriving at this synapse. Imagine putting out one's hand and touching a hot object or a prick from a thorn. The arm is drawn back very fast before the brain has really appreciated which sensation it felt. In other words, for example, triceps, pushing the arm out, is switched off, and biceps, pulling the arm back, is switched on by a reflex action triggered by the pain message.

There must be other actions, such as the balancing of the body and postural muscle function, to prevent the sudden withdrawal of the arm overbalancing the person. Almost equally fast, most people will note the problem and make a memory not to do it again—evidence of a much more complicated event than I am painting.

The most important observation, made with PET (positron emission tomography—we are getting very hi-tech) scans, is that if there is a single nociceptor (a pain sensor cell) sending out a continuous stream of messages, the area of the substantia gelatinosa in which it is synapsing becomes increasingly electrically and chemically unstable.

This excitability spreads proximally and distally in the spinal cord, such that the adjacent cells in the substantia gelatinosa also start to generate messages that are sent up the spinothalamic tracts to the brain. Thus, the cortex may well be receiving many pain messages generated in the spinal cord that have been triggered from a very small bit of rather 'angry' tissue out in the periphery.

Similarly, there will be inhibitory and excitatory stimulation to the local motor system, which may account for the hyperreflexia and the giving way sensations that are so commonly observed in people suffering knee problems and back pains.

It also explains why injection of a little lignocaine into the 'angry' site can turn off the whole pattern of altered behaviour.

(NB The books on this subject are written by relatively young people who are not yet old enough to have suffered. I can attest that 'giving way' of the knee is a reality, and a nuisance!)

The lobulated 'X' shaped grey matter is grey because of the many cell nucleii. Around it is white matter, white because of the lipid surrounding the axons in the schwann cells.

The sensory incoming axons have their cell bodies in the dorsal root ganglion, outside the spinal canal. There are dendrites that go into the grey matter of the posterior horns and synapse with the cell bodies of the sensory neurones that cross to the opposite side and ascend up the spino-thalamic tracts taking sensory information to the brain.

The Substantia Gelatinosa is the area in the dorsal horn of grey matter where the pain and thermo receptors synapse. The Nucleus proprius, also in the dorsal horn, is where other sensory fibres like light touch synapse.

Sensory messages can trigger action in other neurones, both excitatory and inhibitory, which affect the anterior horn cells controlling the muscles. If a finger touches something painful the limb is withdrawn before the message gets up to the brain; the triceps pushing the arm out is switched off and the biceps pulling the arm back is switched on almost instantaneously. A similar reflex inhibition and excitation seems necessary in the observed knee and ankle jerk reflexes.

PET scans (Positron Emission Tomography) showed increasing instability in the Substantia Gelatinosa with increasing afferent pain sensation input causing increasing response in the ascending spino-thalamic tracts; as a result the brain is receiving pain sensation messages that are generated in the spinal cord.

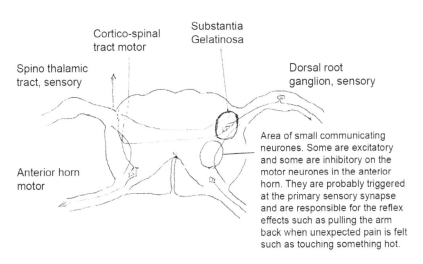

Cortico-spinal tract motor

Substantia Gelatinosa

Spino thalamic tract, sensory

Dorsal root ganglion, sensory

Anterior horn motor

Area of small communicating neurones. Some are excitatory and some are inhibitory on the motor neurones in the anterior horn. They are probably triggered at the primary sensory synapse and are responsible for the reflex effects such as pulling the arm back when unexpected pain is felt such as touching something hot.

Fig 39 Cross section of the spinal chord

Understanding this mechanism is key to managing orthopaedic patients' pains; the simple act of switching off the overactive nociceptor with local anaesthetic immediately stops the generation of these additional pain messages. It takes the cortex a few moments to accept this, and the patient displays a searching behaviour to sense if the pain has really disappeared. And then, surprisingly, they seem to behave much more normally. Indeed, removal of their trigger, and the great majority of these patients go straight back to normal life and work, even if it was a work-related injury.

> I had two industrial accident cases with thoracic injuries. Malingerers both? One was tipped into and churned in an industrial-sized concrete mixer; the other, I am not sure. They presented, off work of course, with crippling pains in their chest wall. Careful infiltration of local anaesthetic and steroid into their respective 'hotspots', both at the level of the pleura–possibly representing scarring at this level–completely cured their problems and both went off back to work–to the chagrin of the union representative, I suspect.

Clinician, until these secondarily generated pain messages are switched off, it is difficult to determine by clinical examination the prime cause of pain. The clinical examination of these trigger-point generated pains have characteristics but they are not those of the classical textbook teachings. They are not difficult to recognise once one has thought of it.

These observations are germane to knee pain when one is dealing with a neuroma but also apply to back pains and whiplash injury. Modern orthopaedics should be about managing patients' pains, however bizarre. It needs the clinician to think about the possibilities, which is not always that easy if they have never seen a case.

> I had a man who had been injured on the medial side of his right knee and had a hypersensitivity in his scar to the point that he was being handed around clinicians as a malingerer and his marriage was in real danger. It was his emotional attitude to not being able to play soccer with his boy that caught my attention. (Soccer and family to Italians are paramount.)
>
> He had a hypersensitive spot in the scar and after some persuasion permitted a little lignocaine to be infiltrated. Once the hypersensitivity was relieved, he acquiesced to the suggestion of surgical excision, which for some reason I did under local anaesthetic. It involved excising a little bit of joint capsule, so was more uncomfortable than I had intended. A couple of weeks later all was forgiven. A sensible family man already returned to work and playing soccer with his son presented for removal of his sutures accompanied by a smiling wife.

Chapter 15

The Mechanisms of Extension of the Knee

Straightening of the knee is done by a number of mechanisms.

1. The most obvious is the contraction of the powerhouse quadriceps, specifically the vastus lateralis, the intermedius and the vastus medialis. (NB To me the vastus medialis oblique is a separate muscle. The VMO is primarily a steering muscle in my view. It is not designed as an extensor, nor as a powerhouse muscle.)
2. Another mechanism—and in life the most important mechanism of extension—is a functional one that only occurs during movement: the soleus muscle of the calf.
3. The gluteus maximus, which extends the hip.

In walking, after heel strike the foot tends to flatten onto the ground. This is a passive movement at the ankle joint, probably controlled by the tibialis anticus in an eccentric manner, that is paying out under load rather than pulling in. (When the power of L5 is gone, the foot flaps a bit: a foot drop.) The momentum of the body's trunk continues forwards. The pelvis pushes the femur forwards and the knee pushes the tibia forwards over the ankle, the foot now pressed to the ground through the ankle.

The most important muscular effort to straighten the knee is made by the soleus of the calf. It contracts when the ankle is at 90 degrees and prevents further dorsiflexion of the ankle joint. By preventing flexion and holding the foot out at 90 degrees to the tibia, the tibia is prevented from collapsing forwards. The momentum of the body carries the pelvis and the top end of the femur forwards over the locked ankle and tibia and thus causes the knee to straighten.

(This used to be one of the 'trick' questions in the multiple-choice questions on orthopaedic exams; they were interested in just how much one had read.)

As the knee straightens and the hip extends, the fascia lata is lengthened. This structure helps stabilise the quads, which are, in walking, only really flicking the lower leg forwards and contracting enough to prevent collapse of the knee.

This mechanism of knee straightening is most apparent in walking. The evidence is there to see in an older person's legs, particularly in an active, tall, elderly woman. She will probably have quite well-muscled calves, but her thighs will have lost much of their youthful muscle bulk. This is because she does not need the degree of quadricep power for walking that was necessary when she was in her running and jumping youth.

It is also the explanation for knee extension in those people who have lost quadriceps due to disease or trauma, such as polio or muscular dystrophies, when they can walk quite well if the ankle is fused.

The same mechanism is used in the application of an AFO (ankle foot orthosis) for a foot drop or paralysis. It keeps the foot up to prevent tripping during swing phase and extends the knee during stance phase of walking.

After jumping off a boat one February I avulsed my quadriceps from my patella. The agent had fallen into 18ft of seawater. I was able to straighten my knee by pushing down with the ball of my foot sufficiently to haul him out of the water and walk the 200 yards to the dockside office.

The gluteus maximus (the buttock muscle) pulls the femur backwards. If the foot is planted and the femur is pulled backwards, the knee will extend. This was a contribution to sprinting that was demonstrated by the training of Ben Johnson—maximum flexion of the hips and then extension, but only as far back as the hip.

We are now bordering on the styles of running and sprinting, which I shall leave to the coaches: long vs. short strides, high lifting of the knees, pushing or pulling ... I was made to do deep, one-legged squats to improve my speed, an exercise also used by the French downhill ski team. Arms out sideways, one leg held out in front and make a deep squat on the other leg. My routine was 15 squats three times on each leg every night. The muscle that got the most fatigued was the gluteus maximus in my buttocks. But importantly, one must work on strengthening the VMO as part of the training routine.

I had big bulky 'linebackers' from North American football working hard on strengthening their powerhouse muscles and getting painful knees. Instruction in re-educating their VMO function cured their problems.

Chapter 16

Movements and Functions: Considerations in Human Knees

Flexion and extension

The movements between the femur and the tibia are quite complicated and are not simply those of a hinge in a single plane. The elbow functions as a hinge, and so does the knee in many quadruped animals. The human knee certainly bends and extends, but there is also rotation about the long axes of the femur and tibia, as for example when we turn off a planted foot to one side or the other. There is also a forward and backward displacement of the bones relative to each other, known as 'rollback' to the folk in the know. The muscles have evolved to accommodate and control all these concomitant movements.

Rollback

The radius of curvature of the femoral condyles becomes shorter the more posteriorly it is measured; the medial condyle is slightly different to the lateral in shape. The axis of the rotation in the coronal plane (looking at it from the side) moves. The point of maximum contact between the femoral condyle and the tibial plateau moves backwards with increasing flexion.

The advantage is that the lever arm used by the quadriceps to straighten the knee changes in relation to the radius of the joint. It is longer when the knee is bent, and therefore helps the muscles overcome the load and straighten the limb for less effort. It has a beneficial massaging effect on the hyaline cartilage, which helps chondrocyte nutrition.

The Maquet procedure was to simply elevate the tibial tubercle to benefit from the increased length of the lever arm. I combined it with an Elmslie-Trillat realignment, where the tibial spine is swung medially, exposing cancellous bone under the lateral tibial plateau. A block of bone can be harvested. The height should be no more than 1cm in my experience (see Fig 51, page 168, and the Appendix).

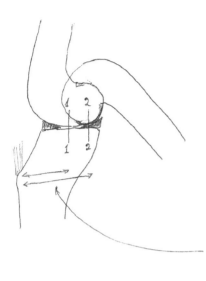

Showing 'Rollback'

Note:

• that the point of load between the tibia and the femur moves backwards with flexion.

• that at full flexion the point of load has moved to position '2' where the load is being transferred through the thin posterior part of the medial meniscus.

• that the length of the lever arm between the tibial tubercle, the insertion of the quadriceps tendon and the point of loading increases with flexion.

Fig 40 Rollback

There is a downside to rollback, and that is that the point of maximum load moves backwards onto the posterior part of the meniscus, particularly in the medial compartment. A little rotation in full flexion, and with pressure, is a potent cause for meniscal damage.

It is the fact that the femoral condyle, particularly the medial one, has rolled onto the thin posterior part of the meniscus in flexion that predisposes to meniscal tearing. As the load is applied through the meniscus, the meniscus gets crushed between the bones and can split. In youth, load with rotation causes the bucket-handle-type tears and the parrot-beak tears. The more flexed the joint, the further back the femoral condyle and the more peripheral the tear. In older people, particularly men, the loading causes more crushing, and stellate or horizontal tearing results.

Rotation

There is a rotary movement in the long axis of the leg. In an intact knee the axis of this movement is between the femoral condyles, and controlling this is a function of the tibial spines and the cruciate ligaments.

As the knee drops into full extension and unsupported at rest, the tibia rotates externally. The cruciate ligaments wind against each other. The tibia must rotate inwards again prior to the beginning of flexion. The cruciate ligaments unwind from against each other with flexion. Standing with the leg fully extended and being forced into flexion by a blow is a cause for rupture of a cruciate ligament, as there is not time enough for the derotation to unlock the knee to occur. It can occur in landing with the legs still extended, as in a 'spike' jump in basketball, for example, or long-jumping into a sand pit. There is just not quite enough time for the unwinding rotation to occur.

The axis of rotation in the long axis of the leg shifts from 'A' on the tibial spines to 'B' the medial collateral ligament when the ACL is ruptured.

NB the bones are of a left knee, The plan view is a right knee. Sorry, slip of the pen.

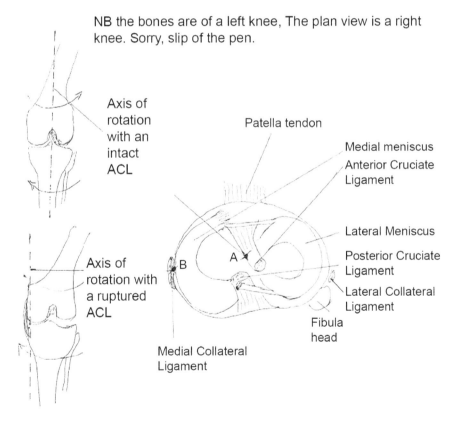

Axis of rotation with an intact ACL

Patella tendon

Medial meniscus

Anterior Cruciate Ligament

Lateral Meniscus

Posterior Cruciate Ligament

Axis of rotation with a ruptured ACL

B

A

Lateral Collateral Ligament

Fibula head

Medial Collateral Ligament

Fig 41 Pivot shift

Rotation of the femur from the hip movements

In the forward and backward (flexion and extension) movement of the hip, there is also rotation at the hip. The femoral shaft rotates inwards as the pelvis is twisted forwards and the leg swings forwards and rotates outwards as the loaded leg swings backwards, thrusting the opposite hip forwards. This is visible in the action of speed walkers, where they exaggerate the thrust of the hip forwards at each stride.

Rotation of the tibia from foot and ankle movement

After heel strike, the foot flattens towards the floor, and as the weight bears down through the tibia onto the talus, there is a flattening by further pronation at the subtalar joint. The axis of the subtalar joint is such that with pronation of the foot there is also internal rotation of the tibia, and with supination of the foot there is tibial external rotation. All of these movements occur with every stride.

(Sit with the knee bent at 90 degrees and the foot flat on the floor. By pointing the foot inwards and outwards, one can demonstrate the rotation of the tibia. By tilting the foot onto its inside or outside (pronation and supination), there is also rotation.)

Long- and middle-distance runners

This subtalar joint rotation effect becomes of importance in the management of long- and middle-distance runners with anterior knee pain. One provides them with medial wedges under their heels and midfoot to lessen the degree of pronation and, therefore, rotation of the tibia each time they land on their feet. (It looks not unlike the Thomas heel for children.) One also trains up the vastus medialis oblique to better stabilise the knee capsule and the patellar tracking. As the limbs and runner fatigue, this can become a cause for their anterior knee pain.

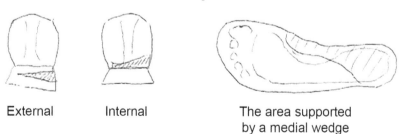

External   Internal   The area supported by a medial wedge

Fig 42 The medial wedge for runners

Cruciate ligament control of forward and backward displacement of the femur on the tibia

For efficient flexion and extension of the knee, the tibia and femur need to be held in their fore and aft position, but in a manner that permits controlled rollback. This appears to be a function of the cruciate ligaments. In particular, the anterior ligament prevents the tibia from sliding far forwards. The posterior one prevents it sliding backwards when flexed.

The anatomy of the cruciates is more complicated; in effect, the length of the fibres varies so that as the angle of flexion of the knee changes, different bits of the ligaments come under tension at different degrees of flexion. This accommodates the changes in the radius of curvature of the condyles and the changes in direction of the displacement forces that occurs as the joint bends and straightens. When the tibia rotates outwards, the cruciate ligaments tighten against each other. With internal rotation, they unwind from against each other.

I have suggested that in my view the cruciate ligaments are more responsible for the static stability of the knee joint; stated crudely, they hold the bones in the right position when we are asleep or relaxed.

In the dynamic situation, it is a function of the muscles to stabilise the joint.

Modern cruciate ligament management is realising that for most people good rehabilitation of the muscles is better than trying to repair the ligaments. Cruciate ligament repair and reconstruction is a very big and well-remunerated industry, and there will be strong resistance to this suggestion.

(NB Cruciate ligaments do not hypertrophy in response to high usage, unlike muscle tendons, and only a small part of a cruciate ligament is taut at any one angle of flexion.)

Stability from the presence of the meniscus

The presence of the intact menisci (the cartilages, in common parlance) or a good solid rim of meniscal tissue also helps prevent forward and backward movement. The menisci cannot escape; they are buttressed all around by the intact capsule. They are triangular in section and form shallow saucers that deform to contain the curved femoral condyles.

Thus, in the normal knee there are a number of movements occurring at the same time. There is hinging, sliding, rotation and rolling. The menisci are flexible and have to distort slightly at each stride to accommodate the condyle. The menisci also act as cushions transferring the load from the knuckle of the femoral condyles onto the flatter tibial plateau. They also probably act as 'pad oilers' distributing synovial fluid over the surfaces and aiding chondrocyte nutrition.

The mechanism of weight transfer in the knee

As something of an aside to the lay reader, examination of the quality of the bone of the proximal tibial in a dry specimen of bone shows the structure as a fine honeycomb of minute spicules. It takes very little pressure to crush this in dry bone. The question is, how does this structure withstand the pounding it receives in normal running and jumping, or just walking?

The answer is that it is full of fluid and fat, both of which are incompressible. It is a hydraulic support. The cortex functions as a sack resisting the fluids bursting out. In fact, there is macroscopic[18] distortion of the tibial plateau with every stride, as demonstrated, by Dr Leo Whiteside, using fresh cadaver knees. The menisci help transmit the load from the femoral knuckles onto the hydraulic tibial plateau mechanism. Within the tibia there is a gradual transfer of load to the thick cortex of the shaft of the bone and then into a second hydraulic mechanism at the lower end. The proximal cortex of the tibia is thin. It is really a tough fibrous sack resisting the explosive pressure of the loading, an important point when considering joint replacement.

However, please note that there is a strong contrast in the quality of the cancellous bone, from the relatively soft at the top end to a very hard cancellous bone of the distal tibial. There the bone forms a socket, and the forces are trying to explode it outwards. The bone is very much harder and stronger. This is important to appreciate when rebuilding the distal tibial articular surface after fracture of the lower end of the bone, in particular the pylon fracture.

In marathon runners, MRI scans of the knees immediately after a race are indistinguishable from the changes seen in avascular necrosis (AVN) of the distal femoral condyles and the tibial condyles. This is a rare condition seen occasionally, for example, after high-dose corticosteroid therapy for head injuries or life-threatening autoimmune situations or divers suffering from the 'bends'. In the case of the runners, the changes disappear after four or five days. It probably just represents inflammatory oedema.

---

[18] 'Macroscopic' means visible with the naked eye; 'microscopic' means you need a microscope to appreciate it.

(AVN is more usual in the femoral heads and can also occur in the head of the humerus. The bone dies because something happens to its blood supply and the femoral head can collapse. But it can also re-vascularise given time and rest.)

Recently, it is thought that the heavy training schedules and the matches of professional athletes, soccer and rugby, may be causing the similar changes and that their bones do not quite have time to recover between events. This may be why they tend to have premature arthritis in their knees.

Wolff's Law

This is a radiological sign of increasing bone density under the medial tibial plateau. It looks whiter on X-ray film. It suggests that the medial plateau is working harder and is stiffer. Bone generally responds to load by becoming denser. The 'Wolff' changes are more common with a degree of varus in the knee when loading is higher through the medial compartment. It also means that the condyle bone supporting the articular cartilage is stiffer and that the hyaline cartilage is subjected to more focused loading. This is thought to be a contributing factor in the development of osteoarthritis (OA) in the medial compartments.

The same changes are seen in the hip condyle, with the same inferences that early osteoarthritis is developing.

Persistently symptomatic OA of the medial compartment can be treated in the middle-aged with realignment surgery of the tibia, the high tibial osteotomy or HTO. Some surgeons are happy to do it; other surgeons wait until the patient is old enough to be offered metal and plastic replacement surgery.

I have seen similar changes in the lateral side of valgus knees and in someone after polio and with a very valgus knee. In that case, the osteotomy must be in the distal femur, but realigned correctly the joint recovers.

I was also sued by someone after an HTO when he developed a foot drop. (The foot drop, which implies damage to the lateral popliteal nerve, recovered completely, I am pleased to say.) But the experts examining his knees 18 months and then two years after the operations noted that there was no apparent arthritis in his knees and that function was painless and normal. They agreed that the operation was indicated. (The patient had returned for the other side to be done!) An HTO is a good operation when there is localised wear arthritis in the medial compartment in a varus knee in a physiologically youngish person (40s to mid-60s).

I have also corrected severe varus knees in young people for cosmetic reasons, although one youth had repeatedly suffered knee pain while working physically on building sites during his vacations. The operation was a painful experience; he and the nurses were quite pleased when he went home. He returned to clinic in his wheelchair with a scowl on his face. When asked what his problem was, he got up and complained that his trousers were now all too short! He then burst into a great grin. (Correcting bowed legs should surely be the ultimate aim of a true 'orthopaedic' surgeon.)

Pathological movements

There is a natural range of tissue elasticity in individuals; some people are not at all flexible and some are very flexible—few of us in the UK could earn our crust as a contortionist, for example. There are recognised conditions like Marfan and Ehlers-Danlos syndromes, conditions where there is abnormal collagen and therefore abnormal tissue elasticity. But there are also many perfectly normal healthy people who are flexible.

When the knee of a lax individual is examined, it will feel looser than perhaps is 'normal'. The examiner can only compare it to the other side and also examine the flexibility in other joints, in particular the hands and fingers. In my practice I would pick up a pinch of dorsal skin on the hand and bend the fingers backwards as a gauge of the individual's flexibility. The findings of abnormal movement in the symptomatic joint, ever presuming that you are examining the knee for diagnostic reasons, must be balanced against the findings on the other side.

However, persons with flexible joints can have perfectly normal knee function. The flexibility or stiffness of their tissues is not the key factor in knee function. Perhaps this is a point to again be controversial and suggest that knee function can be 'normal' without an intact anterior or posterior cruciate ligament. It is the dynamic support provided by well-controlled and coordinated muscles tightening and holding the capsule of the joint tight that provides stability.

I had a colleague who must have damaged his knee in youth. He had no intercondylar notch on X-ray examination, no cruciate ligaments in one knee, yet he skied and played ice hockey without any difficulty and rarely had any knee problems.

Post-meniscectomy

Following complete removal of a meniscus, particularly the medial meniscus, there is increased forward and backward movement in the knee. Again, comparison with the 'good' side may be necessary. A good reason to advocate partial meniscectomy is that the knee is less destabilised by retention of the meniscus rim. Indeed, removal of a medium-sized bucket-handle tear leaving a good meniscal rim gives normal knee function. This was pertinent advice in the era of open meniscectomy. Now that most knee surgery is done with an arthroscope, there is a similar focus on removing the damaged part of the meniscus and leaving the rest; and now, with better identification of meniscal damage, when appropriate, sewing the torn part of the meniscus back into its bed is possible.

So important is the presence of the meniscus to the health of the joint and good function, that it is strongly recommended in the case of a large peripheral tear that the surgeon should make every endeavour to reattach the meniscus into its bed from which it was torn. This is even more important in meniscal tears in youth.

> One youth tore his meniscus at the age of 11 while landing a long-jump in a sand pit—forced full flexion and rollback. During his teens his knee occasionally locked, usually playing rugby and high-hurdling. A moment of concentration and he could unlock it with an audible snap and then run as fast as before. At the age of 19 his knee locked and would not unlock. He underwent an open medial meniscectomy. The only finding thereafter was that his medial femoral condyle, on X-ray, was a little more squared than in the other knee. Function was normal for many years thereafter.

Much has been made of the blood supply, or lack of blood supply, into the substance of the meniscus. Healing is said not to occur in the thin part of the meniscus without blood supply; healing only occurs around the periphery where the blood supply is adequate or there is sufficient diffusion of nutriments for cell healing.

Technically, one needs enough bulk of tissue in the bucket handle to be able to completely hide the suture material.

If the suture material is exposed on the surface of the meniscus following the repair and as a consequence is able to rub on the hyaline cartilage of the articular surface, there is a good possibility that the patient will have a persistent effusion in that knee until the material is removed (i.e. a further arthroscopy after the meniscus has healed back).

My preference was to make a small posterior medial opening and to suture with a curved needle, keeping the suture material buried within the substance of the meniscus. Post-op, prevent flexion beyond about 45 degrees for six to eight weeks. Permit full weight-bearing. I did not have to return to remove any further meniscal tears or sutures in my cases, I am pleased to report.

There are anchor devices sold for arthroscopic reattachment of menisci. I did not use them. If they are anything like those devised for the shoulder, there will be a part of the device exposed on the articular surface rubbing on the hyaline cartilage surface and, I suspect, causing effusion during the recovery period.

Polyglyconate absorbable sutures

I speculate here, but there is no blood supply within the body of the meniscus. The nourishment of the cells is only by diffusion of nutrients and gasses through the fluid between the cells. The metabolism of these cells is probably very slow as a consequence. There is no mechanism for the entry of the body's normal cells of repair (neutrophils and lymphocytes) that elsewhere eventually dissolve away the so-called 'dissolving' sutures. In many patients, in well-vascularised parts, dissolving sutures can take their time to go. My wife pulled them out of the skin of my back some three weeks after surgery; painful. I have had to remove Vicryle (polyglyconate) sutures from patients for scar pain relief many months after abdominal surgery.

I am not quite sure I know what it all means, except that when we used cat gut, things seemed to heal. I think 'soluble' sutures is a little bit of a misnomer and should only be used deep in the tissues and not in the skin or subcuticular tissues.

A recent addition to the anecdotes: A 29-year-old female had a bucket handle repaired arthroscopically; Father is an orthopaedic surgeon. Aged 35, getting up from a curled fully flexed position on the sofa and the knee locked again. This time it required complete removal of the bucket handle, which restored normal function.

Passive knee movements vs. active

In passive motion of the knee these movements are controlled by the collateral ligaments and the cruciate ligaments and the shapes of the bones. In effect, the ligaments hold the bones in the correct positions when the person, or the leg, is 'asleep'.

In active motion the movements are brought about by muscle action, and the cruciate ligaments probably do not have a very important effect, if any.

J. P. R. Williams, FRCS, once one of the best rugby fullbacks Wales has produced, was wont to be demonstrated at orthopaedic meetings to show this. He had a torn posterior cruciate ligament in his knee during his playing career. It evidently was not of great importance to his ability to move about on the leg.

In reality, it is the muscles that place the bones where the brain thinks they will do the most good for the movement the brain wishes to make. Instability is more often noted when making certain movements in a relatively relaxed manner: climbing steps, turning on a stair or getting up from a chair. What one individual can tolerate may be a great infirmity to another. It is probably a reflection of the movement patterns we have learnt and how well coordinated the individual is. After all, we each have the same or similar anatomy, but we each move differently from one another. We have all had the experience of walking up behind someone we thought we recognised only for the face to be someone else's.

The purpose of this book is to promote better active muscle control of the knee.

SECTION 4

Common Conditions and Notes on their Management

———•———

These are really notes for the layman to have some idea of what may have been diagnosed or discussed regarding their knee and what to expect. It is by no means exhaustive. There is a plethora of 'medical', as opposed to 'surgical', conditions and managements—pills, NSAIDs, injections and more pills, the province of the rheumatologist—but the bottom line is still to rehabilitate the quadriceps and the VMO as instructed.

These notes are loosely arranged by the age groups affected: adolescents, young adults, athletes and age-related arthritis. There is also repetition and overlap here. I apologise but cannot think of a better way. In clinic, conditions just turn up and one's management is adjusted accordingly, and one is forever having to give out the same messages.

Chapter 17

Origins of Pains from the Knee

The role of the physician or surgeon is to try to diagnose which structure might be causing the pain of the patient in front of him. To this end, the surgeon must 'think of the parts involved'.

Anterior knee pain or patellofemoral pain

This is still a huge problem worldwide: anterior pain in adolescents; painful knees in adults, possibly more common in middle-aged women; elderly jocks who beat up their knees in sports; and overuse in athletes. The common denominator in all is the pain and its inhibitory effects on muscle function and coordination.

There has been much debate as to exactly where anterior knee pain comes from, particularly in the adolescent. Articular hyaline cartilage does not have any pain nerve endings; nor do menisci. Subchondral bone may have a few, possibly around the blood vessels. Synovium (the lining membrane of a joint) is particularly well supplied with pain nerve endings. The joint capsule is sensitive to pain and the skin is sensitive to pain, but neither are sensitive to the extent of the synovium, which is very sensitive indeed!

Early investigations with arthroscopes during the 1970s in young knees were a bit disappointing in that no one could see any very obvious cause for the pain. Some did note that there was some pinkness of the synovium, but as most surgeons used tourniquets to stop bleeding, usually put on after exsanguination (the technical term for squeezing the blood out of the limb), any slight increased blood flow in the synovial tissue might well have been missed.

As stated elsewhere, one does not have to postulate a big bit of injured or inflamed tissue to get a lot of expression of pain; try sticking a needle into your, or someone else's, knee and listen to the objections! Also stated, it is virtually impossible to see the entry wound from the passage of a needle into and out of a knee—even with the magnification of an arthroscope in situ in the knee joint—so it is not altogether a surprise that little or nothing notable is seen.

Joint capsule

This can be affected by scar pain. It also seems susceptible to a bruising sort of ache as a result of direct blunt trauma. By the time patients get to see the orthopaedic surgeon, there is often little to see on the outside. If some time has elapsed, there is usually a slight loss of VMO bulk and, importantly, a slight lag in its function in relation to the rest of the quads when the patient is asked to contract them (QIS). Frequently, the patient can appreciate it once it has been pointed out to them.

Their management is to get them to work hard at rebuilding their VMO function. For most, this is all they need. The quadricep power for the activities of daily living (ADLs, in the parlance) seems to return by itself.

(NB I discussed scars and neuroma above.)

Synovium

This is particularly well supplied with pain fibres. One of its functions is to clean up any debris or chemicals released by damage to articular cartilage. The other function is to produce the synovial fluid in the joint. This fluid both acts as a lubricant and is the source of all nourishment for the cells of the articular cartilage (the chondrocytes). In the inflamed knee some of the pain is from the synovium.

Plicae are synovial structures, really folds, that close and stretch as they are pulled over the condyles in flexion and extension of the knee. They can catch and bruise, become inflamed and thickened and thus become the definite source of a patient's symptoms.

With slightly more damage occurring, the area of synovium might become just a little swollen and enlarged and more susceptible to mechanical trapping or nipping. What are technically described as 'fimbriae' are often seen in a knee with a low level of chronic synovial inflammation. They look like little fronds of seaweed in the joint fluid. 'Synovitis' is medical parlance for inflamed synovium. Removal of these fimbriae with an arthroscope have, on many occasions, cleared quite persistent pains. I have seen what appeared to be small loose bodies attached to synovial fimbriae. Removal cured the problem. And so simple.

I think it important not to be too sceptical when a patient presents with pain and the clinical examination is more or less 'normal'. The actual size of the source of pain may be very small.

(Treating surgeon, please note: Establish with the patient where exactly they experience their pain just prior to arthroscopy, as removing a plica or fimbria elsewhere in the joint may not remove their pain.)

Plica and synovial shelf

There are plicae and synovial shelves that are distinct anatomical entities or folds in the lining membrane, with similar problems. They are synovial, so tugging on them or trapping them might be expected to produce pain or discomfort. They are the lining membrane (synovium), which must stretch over the front of the femoral condyles with flexion and fold on extension of the knee joint. They are rarely a problem in children and adolescents. Minor injury, or perhaps just repeated rubbing and 'twanging' them over the edge of the femoral condyle, seems to cause some of them to become inflamed. Inflammation will eventually cause a little fibrosis and thickening and then shortening, so they may 'twang' more easily. My practice has been to remove them with an arthroscope if there is any suggestion they could be causing symptoms. It is so easy, and many patients are very grateful.

Some plicae seem to be congenital remnants forming an arch or even closing off completely the suprapatellar pouch. I always removed them, to no ill effect.

Identifying with the patient in the anaesthetic room, immediately prior to the anaesthetic, exactly where they experience their discomfort is always important. Pain on the joint line and lateral is not likely to come from a superomedial plica. Even so, their removal does not seem to be a bad thing. It is so simple to do.

Post-op management is VMO exercises and early return to full function. The step-up type exercise is useful for many.

Meniscus pathologies

In the lay world people have a 'cartilage' removed from their knee; they mean a 'meniscus'. Cartilage is a group of specialised substances, structurally similar but chemically slightly different and functionally very different. It is confusing, but in this tome 'meniscus' is a meniscus and 'cartilage', for the most part, is hyaline cartilage that forms the smooth, shiny surfaces of joints.

The menisci are 'pad oilers' filling the triangle between the femoral condyles, which are curved knuckles, and the relatively flat tibial plateau. They also transfer the load from the condyles to the plateaux. Their bulk enclosed within the joint capsule blocks sloppy sliding movement and so adds to the stability of the knee. (Following meniscal removal, one can demonstrate an increase in anterior glide in a knee.)

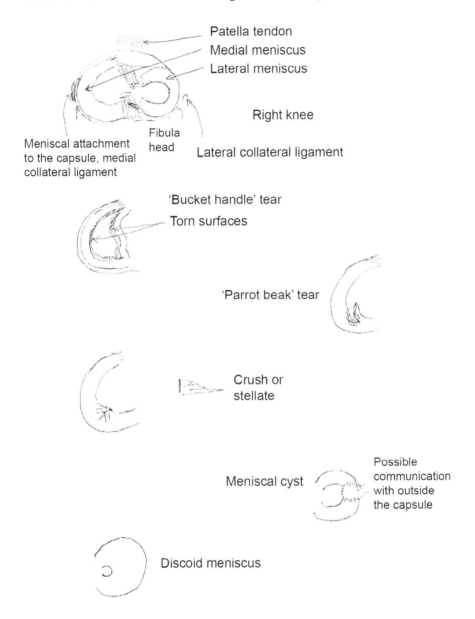

Patella tendon
Medial meniscus
Lateral meniscus

Right knee

Fibula head

Meniscal attachment to the capsule, medial collateral ligament

Lateral collateral ligament

'Bucket handle' tear
Torn surfaces

'Parrot beak' tear

Crush or stellate

Meniscal cyst

Possible communication with outside the capsule

Discoid meniscus

Discoid meniscus and meniscal cysts are almost always in the lateral meniscu

Fig 43 Meniscus problems

Looked at from above, menisci are C-shaped; they are triangular in cross-section, and their flat outer margin is against the capsule. They are firmly attached at both ends and rather less well attached to the capsule; the medial is better attached than the lateral. There also occurs very occasionally a congenital anomaly, the discoid meniscus, which can give problems in youth. Just occasionally there can be a cyst in a meniscus, usually the lateral one.

A tear to a meniscus does not seem to produce pain from the structure itself. There may be an inflammatory response. There is more often the history of blocking, snapping or locking, and although this is uncomfortable and alarming, it is not really an acute sharp stab of pain. It can stop one using the leg. It is not pleasant. But once unlocked, one can use the knee straightaway.

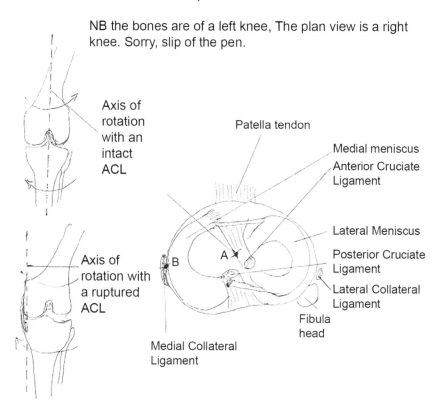

The axis of rotation in the long axis of the leg shifts from 'A' on the tibial spines to 'B' the medial collateral ligament when the ACL is ruptured.

NB the bones are of a left knee, The plan view is a right knee. Sorry, slip of the pen.

Axis of rotation with an intact ACL

Patella tendon

Medial meniscus

Anterior Cruciate Ligament

Lateral Meniscus

Axis of rotation with a ruptured ACL

B

A

Posterior Cruciate Ligament

Lateral Collateral Ligament

Fibula head

Medial Collateral Ligament

Fig 44 Pivot shift

If the meniscal tear displaces frequently, an effusion (fluid) can form in the joint. The knee with an effusion may feel stiff to the patient, although on clinical examination it is not stiff to move. It seems that the proprioceptive feedback messages from the capsule just do not 'compute' in the reflex system.

Management of meniscal injury is surgical. In the old days we did open arthrotomies, a deliberate surgical incision—a hole—into a joint cavity, and surgical removal with Smiley knives. Now we use arthroscopes.

For bucket-handle and parrot-beak tears (see Fig 43, page 121), one normally removes the torn bit, leaving the outer rim of the meniscus. If the tear is peripheral, it is normal practice to try to suture it back into its place, particularly in younger patients. There are various techniques. It is important that the sutures are buried in the substance of the meniscus, otherwise, in my experience, there is a persistent effusion until the suture material is removed.

Post-operatively for partial meniscectomy, early full weight-bearing is encouraged. Limit the range of motion and instruct VMO rehabilitation. Once they are up and progressing, introduce the step-up type of exercise on their stairs (see Fig 14, page 36). Crutches are not to be encouraged in the majority of these patients, although Canadian crutches (a walking stick with an extension that holds the middle of the upper arm) and the bathroom scale trick (see Fig 13, page 35) are useful for some very nervous and sensitive people to get them going!

(NB Some of the proprietary special fixations for arthroscopic use seem to entail material exposed on the meniscal surface, which I think will lead to an effusion in many cases.)

Following repair and suturing the meniscus back into its place, limit the range of movement to 45 to 50 degrees for about three months, so that rollback does not create the situation where it tore in the first place.

(As an extreme example of early movement, a middle-aged lady of my acquaintance, immediately after an arthroscopy in the morning, drove to the airport to pick up an important business person. I do not recommend it, but at the follow-up clinic 10 days later, all the other young sportsmen on the same surgical list were still using crutches.)

Baker's cysts

These seem to occur in the middle-aged who are either having meniscal problems or starting wear and tear arthritis and are repeatedly having a mild effusion in the joint. The capsule at the front and sides of the joint are tough and well supported, but the capsule at the back of the joint is much flimsier and less supported. It seems the capsule gives way and a synovial sack of tissue bulges out. They can become quite large and require a simple dissection to remove them.

Ganglion

Ganglia are closed cysts produced by the build-up of joint fluid produced by rests of cells[19] that are not in communication with a joint. These do occur around the knee, usually singularly in among the hamstring tendons. Like ganglia elsewhere, remove them and get on with life.

Meniscal cysts seem to be related to the ganglion pathology and sometimes they communicate. Suggested treatment would be arthroscopic removal and occasionally dissection to remove the extra articular bit.

Speed of muscle-wasting

An important observation in the days of open arthrotomies was that the amount of quadricep muscle-wasting was considerable and rapid, particularly after a medial side incision. It seems that the medial quadrant is the most susceptible to pain. Once the pain goes, the bulk of the muscles recover. I have measured this in patients on occasion to demonstrate to junior doctors one of the effects of pain. Pain-inhibition wasting seems different to the wasting of disuse. It is more rapid and may have something to do with the substantia gelatinosa and the spinal reflex control of movement. (Those were the days of the surgical firm, when we all trooped around together daily and looked after the same group of patients, and the juniors could be present all the time to learn 'stuff'. UK politicians, please note.)

As a corollary, the least painful place to put a needle into a knee for aspiration, drainage or injection is the upper outer area. Push the patella

---

[19] A collection of cells that have developed not quite in the right place. They are more common in young people.

laterally and pass the needle under the patella. Be kind and use a drop of local.

Scar pain: skin, capsule or synovial and neuromas

These are special cases, but not that uncommon in my experience. They are something to think about. Neuroma pain is particularly intense, almost like an electric shock, and neuroma sufferers become a bit bizarre in their personalities and presentations. I find it interesting that once one numbs or excises the little bit of tissue in which resides their source of pain, they almost immediately become normal! Do not expect to see the neuroma, nor even expect the histologist to find it. They are microscopically small in a much bigger piece of tissue.

There is a sensory nerve that runs down the inside of the thigh and the knee and over the medial side of the shin: the saphenous nerve. There is a well-known branch called the infrapatellar branch that supplies the outer side of the shin. This nerve is at risk from trauma and from injudicious use of the scalpel.

I have seen cases where the nature of the pain seemed to be of a neuroma origin: that is, a very intense, almost electric-shock sensation and very sensitive to even light touch. Usually, there is a scar from a previous injury or surgery, and the hypersensitivity develops in the scar tissue often in the skin or the capsule, and not simply in the synovium. These people have often been bounced around the system but are actually quite easy to treat, providing one thinks of and makes the correct diagnosis and has the technical skill to be able to accurately localise the source of pain. Small injections of local anaesthetic must be able to completely numb the sensation. (A couple of drops slipped into the 'hotspot'.)

Often these patients have been seen by quite a few doctors who have been unable to help them. They may well have been to pain clinics. Often they have just lived with the pain for years. These patients usually need a little persuading that their pain can be relieved and can be quite resistant to the idea of injection of even a very small amount of lignocaine. When the pain goes, it is then possible to show them that one can relieve them of it permanently.

Of interest, if one excises a neuroma, it does not come back, even though you must have cut the nerve again.

1. *In my practice I would initially use a very fine needle, a 25- or even a 29-gauge, and 1% or 2% concentration of lignocaine and just ease no more than a drop into the dermis initially. Then, as the recipient realises that the pain is numbed, I would advance the needle, injecting very slowly until I had control over a bigger area and ultimately the neuroma site, the 'hotspot'. Just a couple of drops of lignocaine in the right place is enough to numb a neuroma. Identify it and convince the patient that something can be done.*

2. *There is a stupid myth taught that one should not inject through an advancing needle for fear of injecting into a blood vessel. One sees needles being shoved in and jiggled about in a nervous patient without any local anaesthetic being injected. This is very poor technique. It hurts and increases the anxiety level of an already very nervous person.*

3. *True, injection of a big bolus of lignocaine directly into a vein, such that it can get back to the heart, does risk causing cardiac slowing and even arrest. I would say that if the practitioner is that clumsy and lacking in knowledge and skill, they really should not be in practice at all! (I seem to remember that it takes over 20 ml of 1% lignocaine to slow ventricular arrhythmia, so it would require more to stop the heart.)*

At surgery I usually asked the anaesthetist to lightly sedate the patient and then re-identify the site and level within the tissues—skin, subcutaneous fat, scar, capsule, muscle sheath, etc.—and again remove the pain with a small quantity of local anaesthetic in a fine needle, reassuring myself and the patient before they went to sleep. Then under anaesthesia I excised the tissue quite generously. I may have made some form of subcutaneous sliding graft to fill the space and close the skin. The patient had to wake with no pain, so I used small quantities of lignocaine, which will wear off quite quickly, not Marcaine, which can last for about 16 hours and burns for many seconds after injection.

Example patients (cited elsewhere in the text)
I offered the example of the 64-year-old Canadian who had suffered bilateral fractured patellae and rather unskilled surgery to remove his patellae about 50 years earlier and had suffered neuroma-like pain ever since. Removal of his pain-producing tissue, and he was completely relieved of his pains and delighted to be able to wear long trousers and play in the snow again—the first time in nearly 50 years.

There were other men with pain following patellectomy for trauma years earlier. The rehabilitation in these men was to redevelop their vastus medialis function, which, believe it or not, does recover. Impressively, their VMOs could be persuaded to function after years of inactivity.

Another most pleasing case was a youngish, mid-30s man who initially presented for some form of medico-legal reason, having been injured at work a few years earlier. The injury had not seemed so very major, but his personality had completely fallen apart and he claimed not to be able to do anything. His wife was desperate. I cannot quite remember why, but I operated under a local anaesthetic. His anaesthesia was less than perfect and I had to excise quite a bit of his capsular scar with him feeling it. I even had to do a form of Z-plasty advancement of his medial joint capsule to get closure. I was not very proud of myself, but the result was impressive. He was totally forgiving about the pain I had caused. His neuroma-like pain had gone, his personality had been recovered, his wife was delighted, he could run around and play soccer with his kids and he had no further interest in compensation. He went straight back to work.

An elderly and very stoic Canadian Indian suffered an amputation of part of a finger years earlier. I noticed he was being very delicate in using the finger and asked why. He had developed a neuroma in the little scar. Using a local ring-block anaesthetic, I excised the scar in clinic. Total cure!

These patients, once their neuroma pain is gone and they understand the instructions, will re-educate their vastus medialis oblique quickly. One rarely needs to see them again.

I first learned about neuroma pain when working as a surgical registrar in West London. There was a very strange man with dreadful limping after an operation for fixing a hip fracture—not done by myself, I hasten to add. I thought he had a neuroma in his fascia lata repair and scheduled him for surgery in the face of great scepticism from my highly intelligent but inexperienced junior house officers. To my delight and their disbelief, the patient lost all his painful limp. He remained as bizarre in personality as he was before. He happily left the ward.

Neuroma pain is no joke for the incumbent.

Cruciate ligaments

These can tear and can cause instability. They can sometimes be heard to rupture by the patients as a 'pop' and a haemarthrosis develops, which will result in a very uncomfortable swollen knee. More often than not, there is also damage to the medial, or lateral, collateral ligaments, and to parts of the joint capsule. This is usually where the maximum pain is, not in the cruciates themselves.

Management of cruciate ligament ruptures is a subject in itself and still far from settled. Mine was ignored, circa 1965, and only now—well, 20 years ago—did I first notice the limitation on a skiing holiday. I have a slightly limited extension, 10 degrees, which results from the development of osteophytes in the intercondylar notch. There is also chondrocalcinosis on X-ray but virtually normal function.

The instability from a cruciate ligament rupture can be masked: good muscles, good VMO coordination and, if necessary, preventing full extension of the weight-bearing knee with a slightly higher heel. This is the first recommendation for the non-sporty lady (high heels on one's health insurance!).

Having good VMO power stabilises the patella and the anterior capsule and can be enough for good function. J. P. R. Williams, FRCS, ruptured his posterior cruciate, and as a budding orthopaedic surgeon his instability used to be demonstrated on the podium at orthopaedic meetings. He was the finest fullback in Welsh rugby of his generation.

Prior to about 1968/69 the diagnosis of cruciate ligament rupture was not known about. We all played rugby and squash and skied for years with our ACL ruptures and medial meniscectomies. I was fortunate that I had been shown the vastus medialis oblique exercises and that I did not have to carry around a 'label' or any clunking knee brace.

In summary, the latest thinking (2021) is that for most people—the recreational skier, for example—with a cruciate ligament rupture and a stable medial collateral ligament, let the tissues heal and then good rehabilitation, particularly of the VMO, and possibly the use of simple orthotics, such as an elasticated tube support, is best.

For the elite athlete, determine if the medial structures are damaged. Let them heal, perhaps with a surgical repair, and then assess whether with good muscle control they are still symptomatic (i.e. is there an instability they cannot cope with?). ACL reconstruction is then recommended, but accepting that they will probably develop premature arthritis in the joint in years to come.

If the medial collateral ligament is also damaged and the medial meniscus torn from its attachment on the medial side of the joint capsule (O'Donoghue's unhappy triad), it will heal spontaneously but may be helped by accurate surgery. It all depends upon the surgeon's experience and skill, and possibly the patient's choice.

People differ, and what seems to be a minimal problem for one is truly an unstable knee interfering with ADLs (activities of daily living) for another; for the latter, a reconstruction may well be indicated.

The skiing season produces many ACL injuries, and worried middle-class ladies would turn up to my pal's office on a regular and lucrative basis. The female knee is rather more prone to ACL injuries, but she is also more willing to hide it with higher heels. Let them heal. Teach the VMO exercise and ensure they are doing it correctly; rarely do they really need reconstruction surgery, and the attendant scarring. This is the recent message from a number of studies. Unfortunately, there are many surgeons who stake their reputations on being a 'cruciate ligament surgeon'! (And yes, I have reconstructed a number of cruciate ligaments, anterior and posterior.)

Bones

Bone trauma can be painful, but fractures are usually diagnosed by radiographs, CT scans or even MRI scans, although they are not always very good for small cartilage injuries. It is not something that one is really expected to look for with an arthroscope, but eventually, when healed, rehabilitation from the effects of the pain will be the same!

Drainage of an acutely swollen knee is kind; an acute haemarthrosis is very uncomfortable. *(Use lots of local and the upper lateral portal.)* The drained fluid needs to be left and observed. If there are fat globules floating on the surface, they have come from the medullary cavity of the bone and indicate that there is an element of fracture, even if it is not visible on X-ray.

Bones, by the way, almost always heal eventually. Open fixation has as complications non-union, infection and poor reduction!

Before leaving discussion of ACL injury, and seen in late teenagers before the growth plate is soundly fused, the ACL can lift up a piece of bone rather than rupture. It is rather satisfactory, if a bit fiddly, to pull it back down into its bed with a wire passed up from below. They heal well and go on to have normal knee function.

Arthrosis and arthritis: confusing words for some

In arthrosis, a joint is showing degenerate pathology but the synovium is not acutely inflamed.

Arthritis is when the synovium is inflamed with an effusion and a warm, tender, even painful joint.

In wear and tear osteoarthritis there is the real problem of aches and night pain and weather-dependent pains. Often such a joint is almost impossible to move after rest, even sitting in a chair, but once movement has been initiated, the discomfort seems to lessen quite quickly. A non-steroidal medication is indicated and sometimes an intra-articular injection of steroid to initiate the settling of the inflammatory processes.

> People vary greatly in their tolerances to the different oral non-steroidal medications. If one does not work, try another. One normally prescribes them to be taken after food.
>
> I treated two Italian populations in Montreal: the elderly immigrant people from the south of Italy who still held onto their traditional lifestyles, and their offspring who had moved to the West Island. These offspring had also adapted to the North American diet and lifestyle. They were much more tolerant of NSAIDs than those living in a more traditional way.
>
> In the heat of Southern Italy one got up before the sun, had a hit of coffee or similar and did one's eight hours of work before the heat of the day. It was usual to sleep (siesta), after which one started to prepare a big meal to be eaten in the cooler, late evening: in effect, taking on most of the fuel for the next day's work. Some of the herbs and the oil may have delayed digestion. The effect seemed to be a greater intolerance of NSAIDs, which by their nature will have some irritation effect on the stomach. The use of omeprazole to calm the stomach is very beneficial.

It seems that the discomfort of arthritis is something to do with alteration in the venous drainage in the subchondral area of the bones. Owners of such a joint can predict the weather.

> Prior to the advent of total knee prostheses, one procedure that could be used in very painful rheumatoid patients was the 'Benjamin' osteotomy. It is of historical import. One simply drove a wide osteotome across the ends of the bones, about 1cm away from the articular surface, through the cancellous bone of both the tibia and the femur and then wrapped the leg in a Jones-style bandage and a light POP cast. The pain disappeared. The idea was that one had altered the venous congestion under the joint surfaces.

Management of arthritic joints is a combination of NSAIDs, intra-articular injections of a steroid, VMO exercises and discussion about surgery.

Other sources and causes of knee pain

Other sources and causes of knee pain include loose bodies which are lumps of cartilage, usually with a calcified centre, that float around in the knee or get stuck into corners. They require removal. Their origin is more obscure. Once removed, they do not return, unless the surgeon missed one!

There are many causes of arthritis (about 60 for acute and 40 for chronic at the last count) that will usually produce an effusion, which is evidence of an 'unhappy' or diseased synovium working overtime.

Investigation of knees has become something of a medico-legally driven ritual. Years ago simple radiographs, X-rays, and blood tests for arthritis screening, if indicated, and a good clinical examination were usually sufficient, and was how I made up my mind. An arthroscope in an experienced surgeon's hands should be able to both make a better diagnosis and also treat many of the problems, or at the very least help create a sensible treatment strategy.

The investigation of arthritis is within the realm of the rheumatologist or the diligent orthopaedic specialist (in Canada, for example, the distances were such that one had to be a bit more of a jack of all trades). This includes blood tests for specific diseases, aspiration of the joint fluid, which is sent off for microscopic examination for crystals, and other chemical tests, all of which taken together should lead to a diagnosis. Management will include appropriate medications, possible surgery and rehabilitation exercises—the VMO exercise in particular, as it is isometric (i.e. it can be done without painful movement).

The medico–legal world requires an MRI scan at the very least! This is much beloved in the private sector, as it is very flattering to the patient and quite profitable. In the public sector it is just another expense. But an MRI is only a test and really is only a way of reassuring, or confusing, all concerned. The problems they raise are:

- the incidences of missed pathology by poor clinical skills
- that MRI scans cannot 'see' hyaline cartilage damage
- overdiagnosis, which leads to iatrogenic alarm

The legal world has much to be embarrassed about. Most of the synovial causes for knee pain will not show up on a standard MRI. The mechanical causes are easily diagnosed clinically and with simple X-rays.

If there is fluid in the joint, the interior is 'unhappy'. If it persists despite good rehabilitation and correct medical management, such as the use of oral non-steroidal anti-inflammatory medication and/or the occasional intra-articular injection of an anti-inflammatory steroid, 'Scope it!' says I.

These patients have pain. Pain will have its inhibitory effect on muscle function, so part of the rehabilitation process must include VMO rehab. And what is left?

Bone pain

This is really a subject in itself: fractures; infection (osteomyelitis), rare; tumours, even more rare. From the point of view of this book—rehabilitation—the same principles apply.

Children presenting with 'knee pain'

In the young child—from toddler onwards—who complains of knee pain or anterior thigh pain, one must examine the hips. Pathology in the hip can cause a radiation of pain to the knee area. (It can in adults too, but arthritis in the elderly is a slightly different fish.)

The explanation is that one principle of anatomy is that the capsule of a joint is supplied by the same segmental nerves as the prime movers of the joint. The nerves to the front of the hip capsule are the same spinal levels as the nerves to the thigh skin and the muscles.

> (Shoulder surgeons, neurologists and cervical spine surgeons, please note that the same principle applies to rotator cuff inflammatory disease, which can present as pain in a C6 radiculopathy distribution, over the deltoid and the forearm to the base of the thenar eminence. I have seen many such patients referred after extensive, sophisticated, negative cervical investigations (including cervical myelograms with metrizamide under general anaesthetic).
>
> In my (not-very-humble) opinion, rotator cuff inflammation is due to repetitive pinching of cuff tissue and circulation cut-off during the hours of the night by distortion of the relaxed shoulder girdle during sleep. On a firm surface, this distortion is greater and is the root of the problem. Eventually, an inflammatory response is triggered quite locally in the affected area of the cuff. The pain irradiates accordingly (see 'Derivative information can be dangerous' in Chapter 4, p10).
>
> The firm, hard orthopaedic bed, 'good for the back', was a misunderstanding. Spinal fracture and paralysis below the level was a death sentence prior to 1948: deep pressure sores, renal tract infections, anaemia, uraemia, and they 'rotted' away over four years. Where there were wrinkles in the bedding, the pressure sores were observed to develop within two hours. Matron had been sacking nurses who were 'not good enough' until someone pointed out that the beds with a body on them sagged into a saucer shape, which caused the wrinkles in the sheets. Matron suggested planks under the mattresses to keep the beds flat to remove the wrinkles.
>
> Alas, the message taken away from the meetings was fracture boards for spinal injuries. Stoke Mandeville Hospital reduced the mortality from 100% at four years to under 8%, with little other management than the prevention of bed sores, clean bladder catheterisation and good nursing routines. And the world needed wheelchairs rather than bath chairs!

But you want to read about knees!

Chapter 18

The Teenage Knee (And a Bit Beyond): Conditions Seen in Teenagers

Chondromalacia Patellae

I have addressed this condition, which is probably the most common cause of adolescent anterior knee pain, and I ask you, the reader, to focus on the incoordination of the quadriceps and the metabolism of articular cartilage. I have to say that many of my peers treating knee pain patients seem not to have really understood the implications of what I have said above.

The name literally means 'sick cartilage of the patella'. It was and is a label given to adolescent, anterior knee pain, although not with any great understanding at that time. Unfortunately, early arthroscopists looking into these young knees did not report seeing very much; possibly, the synovium was just a 'little bit pink'. But as so often, they arthroscoped an exsanguinated leg with a tourniquet in place, and it is not entirely surprising that they did not see very much. They could not find a satisfactory explanation for the pain these young people felt. There are no nerve endings in the cartilage—nor apparently in the bone—sufficient to explain the source of these youths' pain symptoms.

Synovium is very sensitive to pain: think pin prick. A very small area of inflammation, the 'little bit pink' bit, would also cause a lot of pain. It should be emphasised that the inflammatory response is the only response the body can make to any insult, injury or overuse, as, for example, mopping up an overproduction of PG and GAG. Just a little increase to the blood flow causing a 'pink' area of inflammation at the margin of the joint surface may well be the source of pain in the young person presenting with anterior knee pain.

Genesis of chondromalacia patellae

Pain inhibits normal coordination. Imagine the surgeon assaulted as above, with a needle into his knee, limping off to the coffee room. His muscles are not working in a normal coordinated manner, and yet the tissue damage is minimal. The effect of the pain leads to poor control and function of the muscles, and in particular the coordination of the steering muscle (the VMO), which is more susceptible to pain inhibition.

Poor tracking of the patella permits shear and underloading on the medial side of the patella and overloading laterally, and thus, in my view, leads to the microscopic damage to the joint cartilage surfaces on the medial side. There is release of more PG and GAG, more stimulation of the synovium, more pain ... and hence the vicious circle of chondromalacia patellae that these unfortunate young people experience.

Chondromalacia patellae is by far the commonest diagnosis of anterior knee pain in this age group. Teenagers grow. It is not their fault. Most, I seem to recall, just want to get done with it. Growth, I believe, is the root cause of their problem. The obese adolescent female perhaps suffers most from anterior knee pains of 'unexplained' origin, but quite normal-sized and quite athletic adolescent females often present with similar anterior knee pain. In males it is less common, but it does occur.

Puberty in the female tends to be faster, the pelvis widens and the relative size of the hip joints are diminished compared to the male. The result is the increased Carrying Angle (the line between the femoral shaft and the tibial shaft) of the female. This, plus the changes in weight at puberty, requires a different pattern of coordination in the use of the thigh muscles. This does not always happen, and the poor child develops sore knees.

Treatment of chondromalacia patellae

The treatment, quite simply, is to persuade the patients that by relearning to use their VMO, by improving their coordination and by regaining the muscle's strength with an exercise they can do at home—an exercise which will give them a fairly rapid improvement—they can, within a couple of weeks, become pain-free, carefree, normal youths with no limitations on their physical activities. The exercise I refer to is the VMO exercise.

It is often more difficult to convince the parents, particularly if they have invested many hours into driving to and from appointments. More difficult yet is the physiotherapist who has not achieved any improvement and wishes to maintain 'face'. Most difficult are the orthopaedic surgeons who 'have always done it this way. 'Doesn't need an operation. Send to physiotherapy. Discharged!'

A word of warning

There are enormous vested interests in the managing of the persistent chondromalacia patient: weeks of physiotherapy; the selling and wearing of braces and appliances, and their manufacturing costs; the carrying of crutches; the application, and the vending, of TENS machines; the use of 'scans'; being the centre of attention; getting off sports; not having to undress and shower in the changing rooms; control of 'the system'.

I remain unrepentant. Chondromalacia patellae is easy to treat if you take the time to understand it and take the time to make the patient understand it. And the nice thing about youth is that they, at least, are grateful. There are no 'Don't do that!' or 'Don't do this!' or 'It might be dangerous' injunctions or admonitions to be imposed upon chondromalacia sufferers. 'Just keep doing the exercise for at least two weeks and then until it is pain free, and come and see me if it starts again.' One might advise that it is something to remember if there are twinges in the future.

I usually saw young people again at two weeks to make sure that they were doing the exercise correctly. Then they very rarely come back, unless out of gratitude! (The description of the exercise is in Chapter 6).

By no more than re-educating the teenage brain's ability to control and strengthen their vastus medialis oblique, they can get permanent relief!

Unfairly perhaps, I singled out the heavier adolescent females, as they are more obvious examples of needing to increase the power during growth in their powerhouse muscles to accommodate the increase in weight. But in all cases, fat or thin, it is an imbalance between the increase in the strength of the powerhouse element without a concomitant increase in the power of the steering element of the quadriceps.

Males, athletes and sports people

There is also a group of young sportsmen who are trying to 'bulk up' for whatever reason; in my experience, they wanted to play American football. They would do masses of weightlifting with their legs, getting massive bulk in the powerhouse muscles of the thigh. But they also developed anterior knee pain. By specifically working on the steering muscles (the VMO) for a couple of weeks, they all become pain free. Note that in the late teens the hyaline cartilage in their joints is softer than in adults, as they still have chondroitin sulphate. It is more imperative that the conditions for cartilage nourishment under the patella are exact (see Chapter 13 on cartilage.)

Growth and coordination

Growth in children does not occur gradually but in bursts. Toddlers' growth is gradual and pretty well all over as they become small and then larger children. There is a growth spurt between the age of 6 to 9 in which we sometimes see scoliosis of the spine begin, although it usually resolves in that age group unless there is some underlying genetic, identifiable cause. The major adolescent growth spurt is in the pre or early teens in girls and rather later in boys. The timing is variable and it seems to be earlier than a generation or two ago.

Interesting things must happen to the control mechanisms during growth. The brain first develops movement patterns and coordination to control the infant body to be safe on their feet; the cadence of gait changes to become more adult after the age of five. The same evolution of control— or coordination patterns—of the muscles of the body have to occur throughout growth. The evolution of the control mechanisms has to be fastest during the puberty growth spurt.

The 11-year-old athlete may be very good—winner of the victor ludorum—but then a couple of years later their star will fade. The brain just cannot control the growing body very well. Parents often notice that their teenagers seem clumsy. They usually are! And this is the reason why.

What happens is that the teenage brain is trying to learn how to coordinate the muscles for the changing shape, but no sooner has it gained a degree of control, when the body changes again. Some may remember Nadia Comăneci, who won the gold medal for gymnastics in her pre-teen body. She never competed to quite the same degree in her adult body. By contrast, Sylvie Bernier, of the same era, won the gold medal in another body-control sport— diving—in her adult body and could compete year after year.

Once we have finished growing, our brains can concentrate on movement patterns to control our adult bodies. Practice of particular patterns can make a difference: piano practice, rugby practice, neat handwriting practice. (Trainees, please note: 'If your fingers cannot control the tip of a ballpoint pen, how can I be sure they can control the tip of a scalpel when you are operating on one of my patients?' I was accused of bullying!) No one disagrees with practising movement patterns. The same applies to the coordination of the quadriceps. (Consider the diagrams of the forces that muscles apply to the knee joint in Section 3.)

In the female the maturation is faster than in the male. Their hips move further apart than in the male. The femoral neck is relatively shorter. Their knees are together. The result is that the maturing female leg is rapidly developing a higher Carrying Angle between the femoral shaft and the tibial shaft, often to the point that a female may have a valgus or 'knock-kneed' knee. (The opposite, a varus knee is 'bow-legged'.)

The power muscles of the quadriceps are attached to the lateral side and back of the femoral shaft in the upper, or proximal, third, pulling up but also outwards on the patella. The patella is attached to the tibial tubercle by the patellar tendon, and there is a big angle in the pulley system, the 'Q' Angle. The VMO is the steering muscle that pulls medially (inwards) on the quadricep tendon, counterbalancing the bowstring effect.

The forces necessary for good knee function change very rapidly as the individual moves about in daily activities. A little pain, from whatever cause, will accentuate incoordination. Incoordination will alter the loading of the joint surfaces between the patella and the femoral condyles. There may be overloading on the outside, lateral condyles, and there may be underloading medially (inside). It may cause shear damage to the joint surfaces. In those cases there will be a release of the chemicals of the matrix of the hyaline cartilage, PGs and GAGs. These chemicals trigger overactivity in the synovium, whose job it is to clear up these things. If the process is persistent, the synovium becomes a little inflamed, and that becomes painful. A vicious circle can quickly establish, particularly, it seems, in the female.

As a right-handed person, I coordinate my right arm and leg better than my left, but the anatomy is essentially the same in both. The anatomy is the same in Beckham's[20] legs, but somehow he coordinates his muscles differently from most of us. Again, most of us have had the experience of coming up behind someone, convinced that we know them, only to discover on seeing their face that we do not. What we have done is recognise their particular patterns of movement.

Practice of movements, be it kicking a ball or playing the piano, can change and improve our coordination. But just how big is the difference between kicking a ball and scoring, and kicking a ball and it hitting the post? The fine control of our movements is very delicate.

The knee appears to be an exception because it is so big, and we associate fine delicate control with our hands and eyes. The vastus medialis oblique (the steering muscle) is only the size it is because it has to do so

---

[20] David Beckham was a very talented soccer player of the early 21st century.

much more physical work correcting the forces needed to lift and move our weight about, generated by the powerhouse muscles. The delicacy that is achieved by kicking a ball accurately or running and sidestepping or bouncing about on a pair of skis is just as fine as our fingers playing the piano well. Just because the thigh muscles are big does not mean that they are less delicately controlled. The implication of the size of the nerve to VMO is that the motor units are small and therefore the muscle is more susceptible to the pain effects causing incoordination. Consider what happens as the dimensions change and the weight changes. The muscles must be coordinated differently. Pain, from whatever source, causes a degree of incoordination, particularly of the steering element in relation to the forces generated by the powerhouse.

(NB This is an underlying problem in all causes of knee pains and instabilities, not just chondromalacia. The VMO always requires rehabilitation.)

Natural history of adolescent knee pain

What happens to the adolescent with anterior knee pain? Many just seem to grow out of it, possibly because their hyaline cartilage becomes more resilient as they develop adult keratin, sulphate-rich cartilage. But not a few, mostly women, go on with grumbling knee problems into adulthood and start to present to the orthopaedic community in their mid-30s. By that time it is their lateral compartments of the patellofemoral articulations that are beginning to show wear and tear type of arthritic changes. Many can respond to VMO training. For some it may be too late for simply instructing VMO strengthening and they may need something surgical as well in the form of realignment surgery. The instruction in regaining their VMO function is very important post any surgical procedure (discussed elsewhere).

My surgical preference was to do a combination operation of raising and realigning their patellar tendon insertion on the tibia, combining the ideas of an Elmslie-Trillat procedure with a Maquet procedure. It is far more elegant and effective than other well-described procedures (see Appendix, page 193).

One Elmslie-Trillat-Maquet patient came to my clinic, which was upstairs from the shopping mall. She was doing the weekly shop and her knee was a little uncomfortable. She was only about five days post-op. Good screw fixation!

Other causes of anterior knee pain seen in youth and young adults

Osgood-Schlatter

Pain in this disease is not strictly in the knee but at the insertion of the patellar tendon onto the tibia. With growth, the dimensions of the limb increase. The attachment of the patellar tendon is to an epiphysis separated by a growth plate. On X-ray it looks to be detached. It is not, but the increasing loads being transmitted through it with growth can cause it to become painful and a little swollen. The management is to rest the knee.

Resting the knee in a growing youth can be difficult. I had a very low threshold for applying a cylinder plaster of Paris splint. POP is cheaper than plastic, takes decoration better and requires a little discipline to keep clean until the next clinic visit. VMO exercises in the splint, normal weight-bearing and a cure can be promised in six weeks. Once growth has stopped, it ceases to be a problem, but left untreated it can result in a rather more prominent tibial tubercle that can distress a girl.

Bilateral cases are about 40%, but once one has slowed the child down with one cast, the other side normally clears up.

Bipartate and tripartate patella

This is not specifically a teenage problem but does occasionally turn up in this age group. Rather than being a single sesamoid bone in the tendon—which, strictly, is what the patella is—there is a separate element of the patella, usually in the upper outer corner. They usually feel a little larger and are more prominent than the other side.

They are of little significance unless they cause maltracking of the patella and lead to discomfort. Simple excision is the treatment of choice. A small incision, and just cut out the extra bit. Post-op the patient should fully weight-bear immediately and be encouraged to regain full movement as quickly as possible. The surgery, done correctly, should not induce much bleeding. Because of pain and inhibition, VMO exercise is usually needed.

It is a condition that usually presents after puberty. Most operations are on adults. Scars on adults do not grow; scars on children and adolescents can.

(A word of caution: one of my less talented juniors did a case and caught the little circumflex artery, which caused massive post-op bleeding.)

Meniscal tears

These can occur in teenagers and are treated for the most part like adults, except that one tries much harder to keep the meniscus in the knee: that is, one sews it back, or even just leaves it there for the duration of the growth spurt. The presence of the meniscus is vital for the normal development of the joint and shape of the femoral condyles.

One case of a bucket-handle tear in a locked knee of a 20-year-old had actually occurred when he was 12, long-jumping. The knee would have been forced into full flexion and, therefore, full rollback and forced rotation of the tibia under the femur. During his teenage years he had frequent episodes of locking but could usually relax and force his knee straight with an audible 'clunk'. Removal of the bucket handle gave normal function for the next 55-plus years.

Almost all meniscal surgery—removal of the torn bucket handle or repair by suturing the torn part back or nibbling out the damaged bit—is done with an arthroscope these days.

Post-op would be VMOs, step-up and normally full weight-bearing. Following a repair, my practice was to limit bending to less than 90 degrees for most of three months. One must not risk the rollback position.

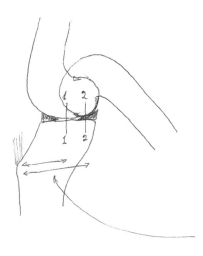

Showing 'Rollback'

Note:

• that the point of load between the tibia and the femur moves backwards with flexion.

• that at full flexion the point of load has moved to position '2' where the load is being transferred through the thin posterior part of the medial meniscus.

• that the length of the lever arm between the tibial tubercle, the insertion of the quadriceps tendon and the point of loading increases with flexion.

Fig 45 Rollback

Patella alta and patella baja

These two conditions refer to the position of the patella in relation to the femoral condyles as a result of the length of the patellar tendon to the tibia attachment. The patella alta looks too high on the lateral view, with an overly long patellar tendon, and patella baja seem a bit too low. Neither is really a cause for knee pain unless there is poor coordination of the steering (vastus medialis oblique) muscle with the rest of the quadriceps.

Plica and synovial shelves

These only really become a problem in adults. It is not often that one has to 'scope' a teenage knee, and in my experience it was usually following trauma. Looking for plica was not really the intention.

I refer you to page 120 where these are discussed. Do they cause pain? There has been debate, but I am convinced that some do, and it was my practice to remove them, slightly thickened or not, as it was so simple. All too often the patients wake and almost immediately say their pain has improved. All they need to do after that is VMO exercises for a couple of weeks.

Osteochondritis dissecans

This is a condition where the hyaline cartilage, for a variety of reasons, appears to break up or at least let small pieces drop off and float freely in the joint. These bits can either stick in a corner to the synovium and gradually be absorbed by the synovium, or they can remain free floating and even grow. In a true case the joint can be quite full of these little loose bodies ('rice' bodies).

The treatment is to try to wash them all out. The difficulty is that some can embarrass the surgeon and get left behind, and one may have to rescope the knee to try to retrieve them.

Loose body

Sometimes a bit of articular cartilage seems to break off and float free in a joint. They may be post-trauma but their origin is not really understood. They can be multiple. We then call them loose bodies. Their cells (chondrocytes) are nourished by the nutrients in the synovial fluid. By the time one goes to look for them, they always have nicely rounded-off margins. Sometimes their site of origin is discernible, but more usually there is no discernible site of origin on arthroscopy.

The treatment is to remove them with an arthroscope and instruments through an arthrotomy on the lateral side of the knee because it hurts less:

day surgery. Sometimes they become attached to the synovium and some are so stuck in a corner that you have to be quite clever to get them out. They are an adult pathology and very rare in adolescents.

Meniscal cysts

These are occasionally a cause for knee problems in teenagers or young adults. To my knowledge they are uncommon and occur in the lateral meniscus. They seem to be a 'rest' of synovial cells that are in the wrong place and produce a cyst – like a ganglion. One just takes them out with the arthroscope, or if they have pushed out through the capsule, one might need a more formal excision.

Discoid meniscus

This is another rare anomaly, when the meniscus, usually laterally, is more in the form of a disc than a 'C' shape. Because the knuckle of the femoral condyle is always riding on the meniscus, it is prone to being folded, and 'clunking' and sometimes tearing. The treatment is to cut it back to a more normal shape arthroscopically. Make it look right and they seem to function normally.

They are rare enough to call the 'boys' in to have a look and at least be able to say they have seen one once.

Chapter 19

Adult Anterior Knee Pains

Patellofemoral

There is an area of crossover from the teenager to the adult, and evidently any abnormality in a teenager will be there as an adult. The difference is that the tissues are also adult—the articular cartilage has keratin sulphate rather than chondroitin and possibly needs higher pressures to nourish it—and it can resist the wear forces better. In the knee, adults presenting problems around the patella are more often under the lateral side of the patella rather than the medial side, but the principles of failure and the management are the same.

I have seen the condition of hunter's cap patella in a number of patients who have sustained quite major leg injuries in their youth—fractures, RTAs, kicked by a horse, chainsaw, falls, etc.—often with prolonged healing. The injuries have resulted in poor or no VMO function and no or a very reduced medial patellar condyle development. Sometimes there is chronic lateral subluxation, or even dislocation of the patella out to the side, and yet the non-injured leg developed normally.

I have mentioned the experiment with chicken bones, some grown in laboratory jars in-vitro. When compared to those left to grow in-vivo, there were none of the lumps and ridges that the muscle insertions had induced.

Most people with hunter's cap patella can achieve great improvement in knee function with the principles outlined here on VMO training and some powerhouse work. If the problem persists, then in my hands a realignment surgical procedure along the lines of the Elmslie-Trillat procedure is indicated, and I usually combined it with a degree of elevation, as in the Maquet procedure.

I have mentioned one extreme case: a woman in her mid-60s whose right patella dropped off the lateral side of her femoral condyle every time she bent her knee more than about 7 degrees. It had done for all her adult life. She remembers being injured as a child. There was no medial facet of the patella, no VMO activity and the femoral condyles were flat anteriorly and the lateral condyle much lower than normal.

I was surprised as to why orthopaedic surgeons had failed to tackle this lady, except that it does require full understanding of the mechanisms of control of the patellofemoral joint, faith in the powers of recovery of articular cartilage, or fibrous cartilage, and the courage of one's convictions to perform procedures not wholly sanctioned by the majority: a combination of elevation of the tibial tubercle, realignment of the tibial tubercle and the patellar tendon, reshaping the patella and reattaching and advancing the vastus medialis muscle itself. It may sound a lot, **but surgery that does not address all the elements of a problem often results in poor results**. The surgery does not take very long. Get it right, and the patients are very grateful.

Plica and synovial shelves

Discussed in Chapters 18 and 19.

Meniscal tears

The menisci, medial and lateral do occasionally tear in teenagers, but it is not very common. It is more of an adult problem. These days one takes out the simple parrot beak and bucket handle tear and the massive peripheral tears one usually tries to sew back. In my hands, a combination of arthroscopic and small open incisions was used. (The presence of a meniscus in a developing knee is important to the health of the cartilage and the shaping of the bones.)

The diagnosis is from the history and a clinical examination, a 'clunk' sensation as it displaces and then an inability to completely straighten the knee (the locked knee), and then for most, another 'clunk' sensation as the knee is forced straight again. This straightening may even require a general anaesthetic.

Having had personal experiences of torn menisci—one on each side— and multiple episodes of locking, I would say that it is not really a pain sensation, but it is very uncomfortable. Once the knee is straight again, it works normally ... until the next episode! The cause is often kneeling or twisting in a kneeled position. Fully flexed, the knee is in the rollback position and the 'knuckles' of the femoral condyles are rolled onto the thin part of the meniscus at the back. The medial meniscus is a bit better attached around its periphery and less mobile. It cannot slide out of the way, and medial tears are more common.

The provocative clinical test is the McMurry test. The knee is fully flexed and the tibia rotated and then the knee straightened. The idea is to use the femoral condyle in the rollback position to pick up the torn bit of the meniscus. With practice, one can distinguish a medial tear from a lateral tear. Parrot beak and bucket handle are the tears of the younger patients. Stellate crush tears of the posterior part of the meniscus are seen in the older age group of 45 plus.

The management is very definitely surgical. In the old days of an open arthrotomy the incision was very painful and quadricep wasting was massive. Today with the arthroscope, one can confirm the diagnosis and remove or repair the damage with much less discomfort and a more rapid return to function. Patients are up and out on the same day, fully or partially weight-bearing, after an arthroscopic meniscectomy. Regaining confidence and flexion may be a bit slow, and these people benefit from the graduated step-up type of exercises. They also benefit from VMO exercise.

Reattachment of a large bucket-handle tear is now usually recommended, certainly in youth. In older folk I do not really think it helps if there is a decent rim left. For a repair to heal, there needs to be a blood supply, which is only present in the periphery of the meniscus.

A word of caution: if there is any suture material exposed on the articular surface, in my experience there will be a persistent effusion in the joint until the material is removed.

Cruciate ligaments

Anterior cruciate ligament (ACL) tears and posterior cruciate tears are a subject unto themselves. Prior to 1970 no one made the diagnoses; people just 'coped'. I deliberately shall not go deep into this subject, but it is interesting that the latest thinking on ACL tear management is good rehabilitation of the muscles controlling the knee rather than jumping to repair and reconstruct. This is a very contentious area, as there are formidable vested interests at stake.

The bottom line in knee pain is always to rehabilitate the muscles controlling the joint and in particular the steering muscle (the VMO). The powerhouse muscles in many patients will become strong enough by themselves. The hamstrings will just string along and always seem to function. I have never seen any real problems with them, even after harvesting for ligament reconstructions. This is not to say that one cannot tear a hamstring; one can, and it is jolly uncomfortable!

Loose and not-so-loose bodies

This is an adult problem, although it may start during adolescence. I have described management above. One must just take them out. Sometimes they hide. Sometimes they embarrass the surgeon, and the patient needs another arthroscopy.

I have seen a couple of cases where there was synovial fimbria with lumps of 'stuff' apparently stuck on their ends. They were getting trapped from time to time. I just snipped off the synovial fimbria and the knee became completely normal. I am not sure if they were a variant of loose bodies or that strange condition called osteochondritis dissecans, where the knee seems to be full of multiple loose bodies. Treatment is to clean them out, NSAIDs and rehabilitation.

Synovial ganglia

Ganglia. These are common, although not so common around the knee as in the wrist and hand. They are closed sacks that fill themselves with synovial fluid. They seem to be little rests of synovial cells that develop without a communication to the local joint or tendon sheath. They can hurt as they grow but usually become completely pain free. They are just unsightly and can be a mechanical nuisance if they grow in between tendons. They may well be the cause of meniscal cysts.

Because they are so common and so benign, there are as many ways of dealing with them as there are authors: aspirate; aspirate and inject steroids; aspirate and make sure they bleed inside; operate, and re-operate when they recur, as they do; or hit them with the family bible! They occur in children and adolescents as well as adults.

Bursa

These are 'normal' structures. They are synovial-lined fibrous sacs that permit sliding movement of the dermis (skin and the underlying supporting tissues) over underlying bone anatomy, over the elbow, the patella, the tibial tubercle and, the most troubling of all, the metacarpophalangeal joint of the big toe: the bunion!

The famous one at the knee is 'housemaid's knee', which is the constant rubbing of the bursa over the tibial tubercle. It swells and thickens. The pre-patella bursa can also swell and thicken. Again, rubbing or banging seems to be the trigger. If they do not resolve with the injection of an anti-inflammatory steroid, it is minor surgery to cut them out.

Meniscal cysts and discoid meniscus

These were discussed above under teenage knee conditions. It is another infrequent condition in which a synovial bursa or ganglion-like cyst develops in the substance of the meniscus. It usually occurs in the lateral meniscus. Treatment is to remove them with an arthroscope and a shaver. In the old days one usually had to do a complete meniscectomy, but this can now be avoided.

Discoid meniscus is rare enough to call down one's trainee to have a look. Management is as above: partial resection, leaving a good thick margin and good muscle rehabilitation. (One does not see the non-symptomatic ones!) Their management is usually precipitated by a tear, and treatment is as for a torn meniscus. If it was an incidental finding on looking about the inside of a knee, I would leave alone.

Osteoarthritis

This is the wear and tear arthritis so common as we get older. It is the basis of a large proportion of the orthopaedic surgeons' livelihood! I describe what can be done elsewhere.

In brief, it usually starts in the medial compartment of the tibiofemoral joint, as this is the part of the knee that carries the greatest load. In the valgus knee it can start under the lateral patellar facet or even in the lateral compartment, although this is rarer. In walking, a normal loading of the knee is about 60% medial, 40% lateral side.

Rehabilitation of muscles. Some elderly friends with symptomatic knees report quite dramatic improvements once they get their VMOs working again. Treatment would be NSAIDs, preceded occasionally by an injection of an anti-inflammatory steroid into the joint to quickly dampen down the inflammatory response that is going on, and then VMO exercises in more advanced cases. Sometimes, surprisingly, long periods of remission of symptoms seem to be achieved by the use of one injection of steroid, provided it is followed by an oral NSAID. Eventually, possible surgical solutions must be considered. Some people are surprisingly non-symptomatic and are written off as bow-legged; others complain bitterly and need surgical help. I do not know why the difference.

When to offer surgery

As a simple rule of thumb, when an elderly person, often accompanied by their family, has significantly arthritic joints, it is usual that initially they are resistant to the idea of surgery. I would suggest to the family that when the patient is noticed to be slowing down their activity because of pain, therefore reducing their fitness levels, that is the time for surgery.

When I viewed an X-ray of my own knee recently—with marked chondrocalcinosis in the mensical remains, osteophytes in the intercondylar notch and a very narrowed and apparently arthritic medial compartment— I was inclined to agree with the surgeon that a new knee was indicated, except that I still find it a very useful organ of locomotion, with no effusion and minimal discomfort however far I walk.

I fear that the 'indications' for surgery are confused with the potential for surgical fees. Reader, beware. If you are developing sore knees, try working on the VMO and persuade your doctor that a short course of anti-inflammatory meds are what you want.

There is a spectrum of pathology from 'normal' to 'outright arthritic'. Age considerations come into the management: a rapid deterioration in a varus knee in a man in his mid-40s, and I would give serious consideration to recommending a high valgus tibial osteotomy (HTO). It should be an elegant procedure and realigns the leg, such that the weight is passed through the middle of the knee. Correctly done, one ends up with normal knee function for many years. But it is usually bilateral, and unless the same procedure is undertaken on the opposite side, the patient looks a bit 'windblown'. Young 50- to 60-year-olds are often candidates for an HTO. For the 'older' patient, 65 to 70 plus (sorry, but some people wear out more quickly than others), one tends to wait until 'metal and plastic' is the realistic option.

I was fortunate to be introduced to the hemi Marmor unicompartmental prosthesis in the early 1980s. It just happened to be the one that worked the best, confirmed recently by a Swedish study. (More about the technology of the polyethylene elsewhere.) It was a very useful step between an HTO (high tibial osteotomy) and a total knee prosthesis. A well-performed unicompartmental prostheses can give virtually normal knee function for many years, which is not quite the case in even the best total knee replacement. There are tricks that one used to deal with the patella.

My expectation for an elderly woman with osteoarthritis of the knee, in my Montreal practice, was to replace the medial compartment with a unicompartmental prosthesis, for they wished to return to kneeling in church and being able to crawl about their garden tending the tomato plants so beloved of the Italian. They were no more stoic than anyone else.

Even if there was some lateral patellofemoral wear, turning over the patella, removing any osteophytes around the edges and often cutting off the damaged articular surface—a procedure we called patelloplasty—could result in normal knee function. If there were some early lateral compartmental changes, we tended to ignore it because following a medial hemiarthroplasty the lateral side of the joint seemed to settle down to normal function in a dry knee joint.

My indications for a total knee prosthesis were really based on the severity of the damage, the physiological age of the patient—not quite the same thing as the chronological age—the quality of the bone and the underlying disease process; for example, almost all rheumatoid arthritic knees need a total joint.

There is or was a place for synovectomies (i.e. cleaning out the diseased synovium in some knees if there is still some hyaline cartilage left), but it is not really germane to this book, although the rehabilitation thoughts are applicable. I can only recall one case of pigmented villonodular synovitis in a knee and a couple of cases in the shoulder. They are pretty rare.

There are 60-plus causes of acute arthritis and about 40 causes of chronic arthritis for the purist to ponder! This is the domain of the rheumatologists.

Arthroscopic washouts

A favourite recommendation of the inexperienced surgeon when confronted with an elderly failing knee. Recent reviews have shown that arthroscopic washouts are totally without therapeutic value. They achieve nothing for the patient except the risks of anaesthesia and wound problems. In other words, they're a complete waste of time.

Chapter 20

Stability in the Knee Joint

Passive and active stability and the role of the cruciate ligaments

The main passive stabilisers of the knee joint are:

- medial and lateral collateral ligaments
- the cruciate ligaments, anterior and posterior
- the presence or absence of menisci abutting against the inside of the capsule

The active stabilisers are:

- the quadricep tendon, the patella and the patellar tendon driven by the powerhouse quadriceps
- the medial and lateral retinacula, strong ribbonlike thickenings of the fibrous capsule that run from the patella to the posterior capsular attachments on the tibial plateau
- the vastus medialis oblique, the steering muscle, which pulls medially and acts directly on the medial side of the quadricep tendon, directly on the patella and indirectly on the retinacula.

Medially, the VMO muscle is enveloped by the retinaculum, and laterally the retinaculum is attached to the lateral side of the patella and so is tensioned medially by VMO contraction. In Fig 21, page 59, the interest is in the lower right corner, the idea being that the curved muscle fibres trying to straighten in their sheath of retinaculum can pull on the medial capsule and hold the tibial plateau forwards.

Please note that the cruciate ligaments, anterior and posterior, get bigger as the knee grows, but they do not seem to hypertrophy to any extent in the athlete, where one might expect them to enlarge in response to a high workload. I am not certain about the collateral ligaments and the retinacula, medial and lateral, of the knee capsule. I suspect that in the skinny individual who gains weight there will be some hypertrophy, although I have never noted that they appear hypertrophied. By contrast, muscle tendons that work hard do hypertrophy.

I would go so far as to say that the effect of dynamic muscle stabilisation on the knee is much more important than the stabilisation provided by the cruciate ligaments. I think the collateral ligaments are very important during movement.

In my opinion, the cruciate ligaments' prime function is to stop subluxation of the femur on the tibia in our knees when we are relaxed or asleep. When the power comes on, it is essential that the bones are correctly aligned for flexion to occur. In the fully extended knee this requires a little rotation and unwinding of the cruciates prior to flexion (i.e. reducing the 'Q' Angle). The cruciate ligaments' size and cross-sectional areas when compared to other ligaments in the body is not very great, and only a part of the ligament is actually taut at any one angle of flexion. One might expect them to be much more robust if they are expected to provide significant function in a dynamic situation, and also possibly to hypertrophy with increased weight and strength. And they don't. (I accept that this is a contentious statement, but I believe it to be true.)

There is dynamic stability and static stability. The VMO is to do with dynamic stability. Certainly, there are many people with a torn cruciate ligament who have almost normal function and who perform many sports to high levels. I have mentioned J. P. R. Williams, FRCS, the Welsh rugby fullback, as an example. He had a ruptured posterior cruciate ligament. As an orthopaedic surgical trainee he was demonstrated at every meeting wobbling his knee about. He was undoubtedly able to coordinate his muscles very well on the playing field.

Prior to about 1970 nobody even made the diagnosis; we did not know about torn cruciate ligaments, so one just had a 'wonky' knee and got on with life, and we all survived.

I had a Canadian colleague who had no cruciate ligaments in one knee and no intercondylar notch on the AP X-ray in the knee. Something must have occurred as a child. He skated, skied and played squash as well as anyone.

The most recent thinking in the ACL world is that for the majority of persons with injury to a cruciate ligament, good re-education of their quadriceps is the treatment of choice. One should only advise reconstruction surgery if they have significant instability during their daily lives.

The body's powers of regeneration and the powers of tendon adaption

Surgeons often use a third of the quadricep tendon with a piece of bone at each end as a graft for reconstruction of the cruciate ligaments. If the quad tendon is re-examined some six to nine months later, its bulk has been restored. One reason why not everyone used this graft was because of anterior knee pain afterwards. Some of this pain, I am sad to say, is as a result of poor surgical technique in harvesting the graft. Training the VMO seems to eliminate this problem, unless the patient (and surgeon) is unfortunate enough to develop a neuroma in the scar!

Following bad stellate fractures of the patella, the bony fragments are often removed. The cobbled-together tendon remains eventually become as thick and strong as the original tendon and patella (between 18 months and three years).

I have re-used a tibialis posterior tendon to re-reconstruct the lateral ligament of the ankle joint. One particular girl was a rather gung-ho, 30ish softball enthusiast who slid into base and twisted her ankle, again! About eight years earlier she had done the same thing, with a resulting complete destruction of the lateral ligament and a persistently very unstable ankle. It was reconstructed by a technically gifted surgeon whom I know well. On the occasion that I saw her, her ankle was again very unstable. I was able to harvest a graft from the same tibialis posterior tendon, which was completely restored in bulk (one takes half the bulk of the tendon split longitudinally for the graft). I was even able to use the bone tunnels my colleague had created eight years earlier! The old torn graft was easy to pull out of the bone tunnels (which might reflect that tendons do not adhere to bone tunnels, cruciate ligament surgeons, please note). She went back to playing her softball.

Extension of the knee in normal walking
It is of interest that the muscle group responsible for extending the knee during normal walking is not the quads but the soleus of the calf. This muscle is said to be mainly slow-twitch fibres. During walking, after heel strike the soleus contracts to prevent the ankle from dorsiflexing, such that it is arrested at a 90-degree angle. The body's mass is moving forwards, and its momentum carries the pelvis and the upper end of the femur forwards over the tibia, which is held perpendicular to the ground. Thus, the knee has to be extended. (This was a standard question in the North American specialist examinations.)

We see evidence of this in the thighs of an elderly woman who no longer runs but walks. The bulk of her calves remain, but the bulk of her thighs are reduced. During light running, or jogging, there is a flick of activity of the quads to initiate extension. A spin-off of this is the problems a patient will have if he is obliged to wear a cast with foot pointing down. This position is called 'equinus' in medicine. All too often I have seen people in this position in error who have great difficulty walking, as they cannot get over their knee—the foot and leg being rotated outwards, as they cannot swing over it.

Chapter 21

Sport-related Knee Problems

There are a number of situations where sport training or performance seems to create an imbalance in quadricep function.

The teenage sportsperson

This, I believe, is another expression of the basic problem of teenage years: the changing shape of the body, the changing weight and the necessity for the brain to keep learning how to control it until the body ceases to grow. Treatment would be VMO exercises and carry on, with no or few restrictions, although remember that the hyaline cartilage of their joints will be softer, still having chondroitin sulphate in them, so it is sometimes prudent to restrict their enthusiasms. Late teens with adult weight and strength—and ambitions—can have sore joints due to overuse. Time is the cure. Focus them on skills and fitness training. But do not overtrain them as may occur in young elite sports people.

The power athlete: rugby and American football

Strange game American football. Some of these youths want to be very big powerful blockers and train like mad to increase their leg strength. They used to present with massive bulk in their quadriceps but not so massive VMO muscles. A short course of VMO training and they all responded well.

Long-distance running

Another strange entertainment: if God had wanted us to run for miles, he would probably have stuck big, hard lumpy things on our four corners, and made it much easier, but he didn't! The chapter on the movements and rotations that occur with flexion and extension of the hips and the rotation produced by the subtalar joints of the foot below the ankle should be reviewed. There is considerable rotation between the femur and the tibia in their long axes at the knee. At each stride there is an increase and decrease in the 'Q' Angle, although the power effort remains the same. As the runner tires, the steering VMO may fatigue before the powerhouse muscles (the quadriceps). Patellofemoral discomfort is the result.

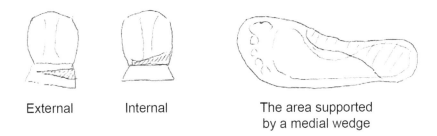

External   Internal   The area supported
                                              by a medial wedge

Fig 46 Runner's medial wedge

The specific management for runners is medial wedges in the heels of the running shoes. It is usual to carry this wedge forwards under the instep, sometimes called a Thomas heel. This prevents the foot and subtalar joints from collapsing into pronation at each stride, and so reduces the rotation at the knee. Add VMO training and the runner is away.

(A 10,000-metre world champion at the height of her powers developed anterior knee pains and was arthroscoped looking for problems. She developed an infection in the knee (the only one I have ever seen in over 30 years of arthroscopy work). It was probably a reflection of the vulnerability of the overtrained athlete when the immunological system becomes impaired. After an arthroscopic washout of the knee, and a course of antibiotics, she was advised to recover and generally become a little healthier, train a little more generally and concentrate on VMO re-education before focusing again on long-distance running. She was able to run successfully again.)

Lessons for the rest of us: overtraining and peaking at the right time are important. Because the overtrained athlete has reduced immunological tolerance, they have to be protected from possible infection. Keeping the VMO in condition helps the knees.

Cyclists

It must be possible to slightly toe-in on their peddles so the alignment of their 'Q' Angle is optimal. I have not worked with them.

I do know that elite teams at the Tour de France have a separate clothes washing machine for each member of the team to reduce the risk of infection.

Sprinters and skiers

Deep squats with toes pointing forwards, bringing the arms round to the front to balance as one goes down, is excellent training for skiers. Work up gradually to 100 per night. Keep the heels on the ground. And for skiers, keep the feet parallel, pointing forwards. When skiing, it really does help that both feet go in the same direction! Just make sure that your VMOs are working well.

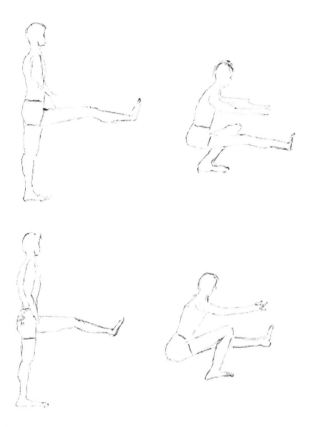

Fig 47 Single leg squats

Single leg squats

For the sprinter, once the VMO is worked up and deep squats are a doddle, squat on one leg with the other held out in front, arms out to the sides and coming round to help the balance as one goes down. It works the balance muscles at the hip and ankle, the abdominals, the hip flexors, the quadriceps and, interestingly, the gluteus maximus of the buttocks. (I used to do sets of 15 on each leg repeated three times every night, and I felt it in my gluteus maximus.) It was taught to me by Bobby Birrell, who was a world record holder in high-hurdles. It was also part of the French downhill ski team's training regimen. Most youth can cut about a second off their 100-metre time with this exercise alone.

Tissue changes

I have had a number of young men who have grown exceedingly powerful muscles but their bones and joints just could not take the forces. Osgood-Schlatter disease of the tibial tubercle is probably an expression of this. Teenage sprinters tearing off their apophyseal attachment of their hamstrings from the pelvis is another instance. The chondroitin sulphate in the hyaline cartilage of growing youth is softer than the keratin sulphate cartilage of adulthood. All one can advise these youths is to keep fit and practise control, but not to overdo it. As they age, their joints will become 'harder'.

One interesting titbit is that the modern professional soccer and rugby players can actually bruise, in effect, the tissues inside their upper tibia and the femoral condyles. This is possibly why they develop premature arthritis of the medial side of the knee. I was aware of the changes in marathon runners who have MRI changes similar to avascular necrosis after a race, but these changes disappear over about five days. It is probably mild inflammatory oedema.

Osgood-Schlatter disease

A word here, as I have mentioned it: It is not really a sporting injury, but it does limit sport in children. The tibial tubercle is an apophysis. It has a growth plate of cartilage (subtly chemically different from hyaline, I seem to recall), and cartilage is X-ray lucent, so that it appears separated from the tibial shaft. After all, the dimensions have to change during growth.

In some children the tubercle area becomes sore and a little swollen. There are not really any radiographic changes. It is very much a clinical diagnosis. Management is to rest the limb, and the best way in a teenager, in my experience, is a well-fitted plaster of Paris cylinder cast on the leg, and strong injunction to keep it clean and dry. Six weeks, and the problem is usually cured. There is a 40% incidence of it being bilateral, but the cast on one leg seems to ease the problem in the other. Apophyses fuse to the tibial shaft at maturity. Untreated, it can lead to a rather large tibial tubercle in the adult, and often the development of a bursa over it: a 'housemaid's knee'.

Ligament injuries around the knee

These problems have produced full libraries of studies: too much for this book. There is great debate as to whether they should be repaired, reconstructed or nursed back to a pain-free status with or without the use of some sort of brace or splint. If you have been unfortunate enough to have had a serious ligament injury—and the common one after a medial collateral ligament is an anterior cruciate tear with or without the medial collateral ligament—DO NOT DESPAIR. The MCL will repair itself. The ACL may become a problem, but the latest thinking is that the early rehabilitation of muscles is far preferable for the vast majority of cases. ACL reconstruction may be recommended for the professional athlete and those with very unstable knees in their ADLs (activities of daily living), but it may lead to early osteoarthritis.

There were a few cases, in my experience, with adolescents, when the growth plate had not completely closed and where the ACL had avulsed the bony tibial origin. One could pull it back into place with a wire passed up through the tibial plateau. Delicate surgery, but very doable and results in a normal knee eventually.

O'Donoghue's unhappy triad

The 'blown knee' of medial collateral ligament tear, meniscal tear and cruciate ligament injury should not be dismissed, but it is not very common. In my hands, I tried to repair the medial structures and to sew the meniscus back if possible. I rather ignored the anterior cruciate, preferring for the patient to repair everything else and regain VMO function.

The modern thinking on ACL repairs is to try to avoid them. Good rehabilitation, including the re-education and strengthening of the VMO, is by far the most useful thing the average person can do. A simple neoprene or elastic sleeve around the knee was all that was used (sometimes on the good knee so the opposition would not target one's bad knee!).

Interestingly, walking in a shoe with a raised heel seems to improve the stability of the ACL-injured female, probably because the knee does not quite straighten in high heels. Once the muscles are fully recovered and the VMO function fully restored she can usually dispence with the high heels! (A nice thought: high heels prescribed on one's medical insurance.)

Note on elasticated tubes and strapping around the knee

They can make the knee 'feel' better, and thus it works better. Just what the mechanism is, I am uncertain, but I suspect that it the augmentation of the proprioceptive impulses from the skin and dermis—a bit like the Chinese burn of youth. The reflex control systems have to 'listen to' or 'process' all inputs, and the discomfort messages are diluted.

I do not think that rings, doughnuts or straps to 'align' the patella are particularly useful. VMO exercises should do that. But there is no doubt that the wimping athlete can improve his performance wearing such a device.

My thoughts on strapping fall into the same category: if it feels better, you will probably use it better, but it is not a substitute for getting the VMO working correctly.

Knee braces

These were popular in the 1970s and 1980s. I think they were over-prescribed, but they looked good. One is not permitted to wear them in European contact sports. At one point, wearing a Lennox Hill knee brace seemed like a requirement in the gym. There was a paper that suggested that using them prophylactically to try to prevent severe ligament injury actually increased the incidence of injury.

Did they do any good? There were some middle-aged jocks who seemed to play better squash wearing them. I think better VMO training might have helped more, but it was always an excuse if one lost.

Chapter 22

Hamstrings: A Note

Many will accuse me of ignoring the hamstrings. These are the flexors of the knee that are attached to the inside and outside of the tibial plateau, and they very much exist; but in reality, and in my experience, they do not cause problems of knee pain.

One can tear a hamstring, and it is very painful and takes surprisingly long to recover. Young athletes can avulse their origins from the ischial spine. There is little to do but rest and wait. Some surgeons use the hamstrings to reconstruct the anterior cruciate ligament. Not the technique that I used; I found that bone–patella–bone worked well. Bone always heals to bone, and tendon does not like to heal into bone. The patellar tendon remaining in situ will hypertrophy over six months, and the VMO can be trained and relieves all anterior pain worries. (The problems of post-reconstruction anterior knee pain seem due to poor harvesting technique and repair, in my ever-so-humble opinion.)

The physiotherapy world works hard with hamstrings. Some feel that the hamstrings need to be retrained when dealing with anterior knee problems; I have never bothered. In my experience, providing that the steering element of the quads (the VMO) is adequately dealt with, the knee function seems to return to pain-free 'normalcy'.[21] This does not mean that hamstrings do not need to be stretched and warmed up prior to vigorous use.

---

[21] I love/hate that word. I read somewhere: 'Normalcy is a vestigial concept left in medicine from the pre-scientific era.' (one 'Wilson', circa 1968, whoever he was). What tosh! Observation is the first stage in the scientific method. Remembering that, art in medicine is the perception and manipulation of parameters that science cannot yet measure.

Chapter 23

Genu Varus and OA Surgical Options: HTO to Hemi-arthroplasty

Bow-legged for many is a minimal problem, but with advancing age, the repetition of overload on the medial tibial plateau can start to become symptomatic, or intermittently painful, during or after exercise. It is a simple mechanical problem. Treatment is also simple: straighten the tibia with a high tibial osteotomy (HTO). It then requires the patient to relearn how to use their VMO, and years of trouble-free motoring can be assured. But...!

So where are the problems? In theory, there is a 'window of opportunity', when the medial compartment has the ability to heal itself. Judging that period requires rather more experience than many surgeons achieve in a lifetime. Actually, in my experience, it is a little wider than many surgeons believe.

First do no harm. Operations and anaesthetics are not completely without risks. Although much of the risk is the skill of the operator and how long the procedure takes—and, sadly, not all surgeons are technically as deft with their hands as perhaps they should be—one does need to be a good 'eyeball' surgeon because despite the various jigs devised (and I helped invent one) to help determine the degree of correction necessary, the time wasted using the jigs increases, slightly, the risks. In my experience, cutting and getting the angle of the leg right depends upon the eye.

A high tibial osteotomy (see Fig 48 on the following page) can be done bilaterally, although it is jolly uncomfortable for the patient. Doing it sequentially requires even more judgement to get the second one exactly the same as the first. I have done it bilaterally in some young people for both functional and cosmetic reasons, sometimes in the face of opposition from colleagues. The patients and their families were very grateful.

For the girls, after puberty and when the growth plates have fused it can be done through a short oblique incision that is cosmetically acceptable (see Langer's lines).

161

Wedge of bone removed leaving
the medial cortex as the hinge.

About half of the head of the fibula
is removed, otherwise it is too long.

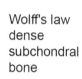

Wolff's law
dense
subchondral
bone

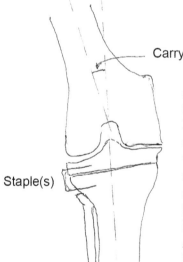

Carrying angle restored

Normally protect the lateral popliteal
nerve. Pass two 'K' wires across the
bone to guide the bone cuts (check
X-ray advised).

Cut with an oscillating saw to remove the
wedge of bone.

Staple(s)

Use step staples to hold the closed
osteotomy. This requires a little eyeball
positioning, particularly if it is a bi lateral
procedure.

Application of a well moulded POP cast.
Permit almost immediate weight bearing
but elevate when at rest.

Normally done using local infiltration with
a Marcaine and adrenalin solution and no
tourniquet. Suction drain through the cast.

Fig 48 High valgus tibial osteotomy

In late forty- and fifty-year-olds I have done it sequentially. One man developed a foot drop after the first one, probably from a bleed into his lateral popliteal nerve, and started a litigation, but his knee became so comfortable and the foot drop recovered that he presented asking for the other to be done. And went on to have good knee function for years.

Baker's cyst

This is sometimes called a popliteal cyst. It is not confined to a varus knee but is most common in this age group, where arthritic processes are starting (i.e. the middle-aged and older aged). It is very rare in youth, where it may be a different pathology, like a synovial ganglion. They are not seen so very often that their management is common place for a surgeon.

It is easiest to envisage their genesis as a low-grade degenerative type arthritic process or a mechanical cause, such as a meniscal tear producing just a little too much synovial fluid. The front and side capsule of the joint is very solidly buttressed by the retinacula, collateral ligaments each side and the quadricep mechanism, the attached medial meniscus medially and popliteus tendon laterally, all of which structures are pretty solid. By contrast, the capsule at the back of the knee is relatively unsupported and is 'lax' in most positions of the knee. The synovium lining a joint overproducing synovial fluid can bulge through the weaker areas of the capsule and then form a cystic structure outside the joint between the structures, usually behind the knee.

The most straightforward line of treatment is a simple elasticated wrap. This slightly increases the pressure within the joint and can help to increase the rate of reabsorption of the synovial fluid; perhaps not quite how it works, but it does feel better. Mixing modalities, NSAIDs and even an intra-articular injection of an anti-inflammatory steroid backed by a course of NSAIDs can hold it at bay for some time. Correction of the problem causing the overproduction of synovial fluid is the real treatment.

If it cannot be controlled chemically or has become very extensive, then occasionally one resorts to a surgical dissection to remove the cyst, but one still has to address the cause of the overproduction of synovial fluid or it will just reoccur. Just occasionally, a large baker's cyst will burst into the calf and be quite painful.

A synovial ganglion can be confused with a baker's cyst, but these are not common around the knee. Ganglia are a problem for young people in their teens and 20s. Excision is the treatment of choice.

Unicompartmental prosthesis

So, as the 'window' closes for an HTO, what are the next options? In my view a unicompartmental prosthesis or hemi-arthroplasty (i.e. metal and plastic), where the bone quality is normally good, is the option of choice if technically possible. (We are talking the wear and tear osteoarthritis here. Other causes of arthritis require different considerations and would not have been subject to a realignment surgery.)

I and my patients were fortunate in that the hemi-Marmor (the first unicompartmental prosthesis) was available. It was made by Richards. In forming and sterilising the ultra-high-density polyethylene (UHDPE) of the tibial component, different companies chose different procedures. Richards' UHDPE stood the test of time. Other companies' UHDPE products did not, which very much skewed the evaluation of the procedure in certain academic quarters.

Also, the prosthesis had two components that mimicked the shape of the femoral condyle and the tibial plateau. Most importantly, in my view, the tibial component was let into the top of the tibial plateau so the loading was onto nature's hydraulic mechanism rather than trying to balance the component onto the rather thin tibial plateau cortex, a cortex that was not evolved to be load-bearing but to resist the expansive forces of compression in the hydraulic mechanism.

On follow-up radiography of Marmor prostheses after some years, there appeared to be loosening lines under the tibial component, but function was not affected. In real life the tibial plateau deforms under normal walking loads (as demonstrated by Leo Whiteside, MD). The original hemi-Marmor tibial component did not have a metal backing. I think they actually performed better than the later metal-backed ones. They never became very popular in the UK but were used in Sweden, who recently reported better results with the Marmor than other unicompartmental prostheses.

There is now a plethora of unicompartmental prostheses on the market; each surgeon probably has his or her own preference and each is promoted by pretty powerful commercial interests.

Our observations 30-plus years ago showed that once the arthritic medial compartment was treated, the lateral compartment settled down and the patellofemoral problems responded to patellaplasty and VMO training.

And therein lies another objection. Too many inexperienced surgeons believe that one can only do a successful hemi-arthroplasy in unicompartment disease. Or that two compartment disease is a contraindication, therefore, 'Wait until you need a total joint!'

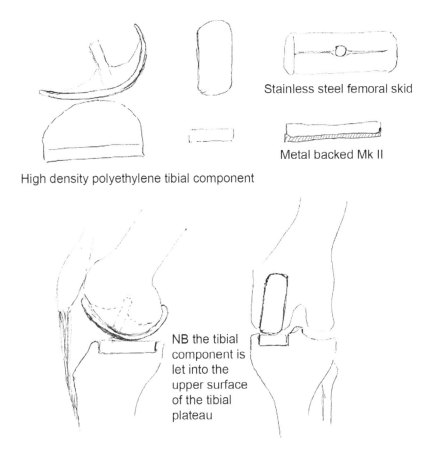

Stainless steel femoral skid

Metal backed Mk II

High density polyethylene tibial component

NB the tibial component is let into the upper surface of the tibial plateau

Fig 49 Hemi-Marmor prosthesis

In a world where the doctor gets a fixed salary however hard he works, why should he push himself? Where 'fee for item of service' applies—North America, Europe, private practice—more effort is made to offer other possibilities. But at some North American meetings, radiographs were shown that did not to my eye warrant surgical intervention at all!

Where does that leave you, the bow-legged patient whose knees are starting to get symptomatic? At least you are now informed and can discuss sensibly with the surgeon you choose and assess if he is the right man for you. The operation of a valgus high tibial osteotomy (HTO) in good hands is not technically very difficult, nor for that matter is putting in a unicompartmental prosthesis.

An HTO can be done through quite a small anterolateral oblique incision that can be very cosmetically acceptable. Long midline incisions are not necessary for an HTO. It helps greatly if the fine osteotomes are sharp! For fixation I usually used stepped staples and a cylinder cast but have also used screws and wire. Tibial cancellous bone heals very quickly. The staples can be left in or removed at a later date.

The HTO window is late-40s to early/mid-60s; one has to assess the whole patient.

Hemi-arthroplasties work so much better than total knee replacements, and to my mind it is the treatment of choice in most osteoarthritic situations. Inflammatory arthritides and poor bone stock does, I am sorry to say, mean a TKR (total knee replacement).

And remember that before and after any knee surgery, working up the VMO function will always help!

Cosmetic and functional considerations in youth

There is a small group of patients, teenagers even, with very marked varus knees. There are also specific conditions of congenital failure of the medial plateau. This is very specialist and is managed on an individual basis. Timing in youth should be after the growth plates have fused.

I have on occasion done high tibial osteotomies to give these young people normal-shaped legs. My colleagues were usually critical, as it entails all the risks of surgery, but the patients and their families were very grateful. They do, however, suffer; it is painful and very disabling for about a month. But they are grateful, as reported on page 126.

Surgery for patellofemoral problems

In my opinion there are two very useful procedures for a number of people, ladies more usually, with lateral patellar facet arthritis: a patelloplasty and an elevation and realignment, the Elmslie-Trillat-Maquet procedure. I often used them together.

The patelloplasty we used in conjunction with a hemi-arthroplasty; you already have the knee open. Patelloplasty arthroscopically combined with realignment is good for simple patellofemoral problems. I was very sceptical of plastic patellar buttons alone.

Pre-op and post-op concentration on VMO exercises goes without saying! This is what you can do to the patella.

To get a good cosmetic result from the ETM realignment does require a little manual skill with a long, sharp osteotome through a small, oblique, laterally placed incision. The bone-cutting and elevation is done

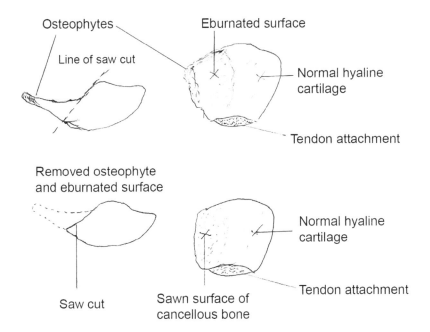

Turn the patella over and cut off the osteophytes and any eburnated bone. One can cut to expose cancellous bone. With immediate or very early movement one can expect the surface to become covered with either fibro-cartilage of even hyaline cartilage. It becomes a hard wearing articular surface without patients complaining of pain.

Fig 50 Patelloplasty

subcutaneously: multiple passes from the side and then gently lever up the tibial crest with the tibial tubercle and swing it medially. The bone block is harvested from the exposed cancellous bone of the lateral tibial plateau. Fixation is with one countersunk screw just catching the posterior tibial cortex. I found it a very useful procedure on occasion.

One lady did come to clinic complaining that the wound was a little painful. 'Would I look at the wound?' She was only four or five days post-op.

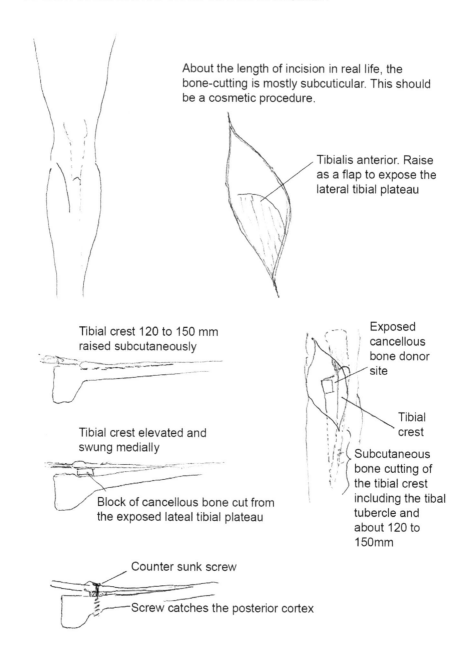

About the length of incision in real life, the bone-cutting is mostly subcuticular. This should be a cosmetic procedure.

Tibialis anterior. Raise as a flap to expose the lateral tibial plateau

Tibial crest 120 to 150 mm raised subcutaneously

Tibial crest elevated and swung medially

Block of cancellous bone cut from the exposed lateal tibial plateau

Exposed cancellous bone donor site

Tibial crest

Subcutaneous bone cutting of the tibial crest including the tibal tubercle and about 120 to 150mm

Counter sunk screw

Screw catches the posterior cortex

ELMSLIE TRILLAT MARQUET PROCEDURE
Elevation of the tibial tubercle with realignment. Usually about 1 cm elevation, no more.

Fig 51 Elevation and realignment of the tibial tubercle

For the surgeon contemplating this procedure, particularly if the lateral patellar facets seem badly worn, do not despair. If I could not remove the osteophyte and clean up the lateral facet arthroscopically (shavers were not invented when I was first doing this), I used to use a sort of reversed Timbrel-Fisher-style anterior incision but on the lateral side. It can be shorter and turn the patella over. I would then cut off all the osteophytes and even smooth the patella's lateral facet to cancellous bone (as per the diagrams). Once one has swung the tibial tubercle medially, there is exposed cancellous bone under the lateral tibial condyle from whence one can harvest a block to elevate the tibial tubercle. I was able to use immediate CPM, which seemed to help the patients gain the confidence to bend the knee. VMO exercises and loads of movement, and they really recovered completely. The joys of healing cartilage!

Knee prosthetics and prostheses

In discussing knee pains, there are people who need to know something about prosthetic possibilities in the knee.

Perhaps the simplest is some form of elasticated tube or wrap, with or without straps, or the popular strapping as seen on the sports field. I have reflected on why they work. I think it may be related to the proprioceptive feedback from the cutaneous tissues, a bit like a Chinese burn one inflicted in childhood. The sensation-sampling mechanisms of the spinal cord and brain, reflex or otherwise, must, it seems, sample every input. The skin contribution seems to dull other sensations.

I am less enamoured with braces. I have talked about them above. ACL braces were over prescribed. One is not permitted to wear them in European contact sports. There was a paper that suggested that those who wear 'protective' braces are actually more prone to injury. I have met some middle-aged squash players who found them useful, but then perhaps better quadricep re-education might have done the same thing.

Over the course of my orthopaedic career there have been many, many artificial knee prostheses. Some are good and some were … dreadful. (One does have to be a little discrete, even old and grey as I am.)

Broadly speaking, there are total knee replacement prostheses, unicompartmental prostheses—in which only one side of the knee joint is replaced—and patellofemoral replacements.

Of the total prostheses there are those that are unstabilised, relying on good muscles and ligaments and capsule, and there are a variety of stabilised prostheses that try to take over where ligaments are missing, more usually used in revision surgery or the very weak bone in something like rheumatoid. In this you, the patient, are going to have to trust your surgeon. He will do a better job with the ones he is used to using.

Metallurgy—stainless steel 316 in implants—is usually used for the bearing surfaces. It has stood the test of time. Titanium is better accepted by the body's tissues, but it makes for poor bearing surfaces. It is sometimes used to support UHMWPE (see below) plastic bearing surfaces, as bone rather likes titanium and 'biological' fixation can be achieved.

Regarding ceramics, various forms have been used and they make very low-friction articular surfaces. I do not know of their use in knee joints, but they are excellent in hip joints.

Polyethylene, then high-density polyethylene and now ultra-high molecular-weight polyethylene (UHMWPE) is used for one bearing surface, almost always against stainless steel or ceramic, in total and hemi-arthoplasties. It works well but ... and there are a number of interesting 'buts'.

The granules of the raw polyethylene were produced globally by only a few suppliers who sold in bulk to the prosthetic manufacturers. The prosthetic manufacturers do not, or did not, always treat it in the same way. As the problems became evident, they changed their procedures used to mold their particular prosthesis. I was fortunate to use the hemi-Marmor, a unicondylar prosthesis made by Richards. Richards' high-density polyethylene in the 1980s was durable and stood the test of time. Other well-known companies produced hemi-arthroplasties but used different manufacturing and sterilisation processes, and the resultant high-density polyethylene did not stand up. Sterilisation techniques seemed to be the biggest problem. The hemi-arthroplasty as a procedure got a bad reputation, not because the procedure is bad but because of the high failure rate of the plastic produced by one of the world's leading producers (names withheld to protect the guilty, or perhaps just unfortunate; they have tried hard to eliminate the problems). One also had to be aware that surgeons were reluctant to admit that their surgical skill, or lack of it, was why some procedures were slow to be accepted.

Hemi-arthroplasties also suffered because of the desire to use jigs to site them, and the jigs required the cortex of the tibial plateau to sit the prosthesis on. As explained elsewhere, the mechanism of load transfer through the plateaux is hydraulic, and not via the cortex. I think that the surgeon needs the confidence to be able to 'eyeball' the placement of a unicompartmental prosthesis. The hemi-Marmor was let into the tibial plateau and sat on the cancellous hydraulic mechanism. On a review X-ray it often appeared loose, as a radiolucent line could often be seen, but it seemed to go on functioning very well.

Since those early years of development, it has been shown that different pressures, different temperatures and different sterilisation techniques can all affect the quality of the final high-density polyethylene. Radiation, for example for sterilisation, alters the cross-link structure of the plastic. In modern practice, UHMWPE (ultra-high molecular-weight polyethylene) is much improved. Incorporating an oxidant like vitamin E can apparently increase its durability.

One not-so-small problem with evaluating things like total joints is that you put them in and then have to wait 10, 15, 20 or more years to know which ones do best. It can be difficult to separate which factor is responsible for which improvement. Getting one's name onto a prosthesis was not only flattering but financially rewarding. During my career, it seemed that too many people were experimenting with too many different designs. One knee prosthesis got up to about mark 10 before people gave up on it.

What was interesting for me, working to one side but quite close to the academic world, was that those models that fairly closely mimicked the anatomy of the femoral and tibial condyles seemed to work best. Being too clever or simplistic in the designs tended not to be as functional as nature's own design.

Size in knee-joint prosthetics has two important aspects. The condyles need to be about the same size as the natural ones being replaced to fit into the capsule, but there is also the important thickness of the joint surfaces: how far the bones—femur and tibia—are held apart by the prosthesis. If the surgeon made the error of overstuffing the joint with too thick a prosthesis, the patients had problems. If the surgeon put in a prosthesis that was a little too thin or cut off a little too much bone, such that the joint was a little sloppy, the patients were actually much happier. With good rehabilitation of their quadriceps and VMO, the patients were functionally able to mask any instability that clinical examination might seem to demonstrate. Tight, overstuffed knees do badly.

The management of the patellofemoral joint is also much debated. Some surgeons always place a patellar button (a plastic replacement surface for the patella) when doing a total knee replacement; some never place a patellar button. I did both in total joints, but I am not certain which was correct.

In unicompartmental replacements I never placed a patellar button, even if the lateral patellofemoral joint was damaged. I almost always performed some degree of patelloplasty: that is, turning the patella over and trimming its articular surfaces to fit. Most usually, it is a rather worn lateral surface, with osteophytes forming a sort of hook preventing the patella moving medially. Even removing all hyaline cartilage down to cancellous bone seemed to produce a good pain-free patellofemoral articulation, provided that immediate movements were instigated.

Patelloplasty was not in common orthopaedic practice, but I strongly recommend it to any surgeon who professes to be an expert knee surgeon. And to the patient: ask the bugger, and if he does not know what you are talking about, change surgeons.

Aseptic loosening and revision

There is a condition called aseptic loosening that was seen in early total joint replacement patients. Sepsis (i.e. infection) was always a concern when a foreign body was implanted into a patient. These joints looked a bit like an infection. But there was no infection. There was bone reabsorption, and the prosthesis became completely loose. There was a thick, juicy membrane with masses of giant cells lining the cavity that could be scraped off. Histology eventually elucidated the problem.

The older high-density polyethylene wore and microscopic bits of plastic sloshed around in the joint fluid. One type of cell in synovium is responsible for mopping up debris. The cells would engulf the plastic fragments, like amoeba, and try to digest it, except that they were not able to digest polyethylene. They coalesced into giant cells, with multiple nuclei that poured our lytic enzymes that did not affect the plastic but lysed away the bone. The trigger was the plastic debris.

(NB Plastic problems in the oceans of the world had not then been appreciated, but it is the same phenomenon: biological systems cannot degrade most plastics.)

Management of an aseptic loosening is surprisingly easy. Open the joint, remove the old prosthesis and any cement, then scrape out all the membrane and debris. Open into the marrow cavity[22] and using quite a lot of bone graft, put in a new prosthesis—if possible, without using more cement. I needed two, occasionally three, femoral heads of graft bone for a revision knee replacement, particularly for the Sheehan. One I halved and

---

[22] Part of the trigger to bone fracture healing and callus formation is that at the fracture site the electropotential difference in bone between the endosteum and periosteum is disturbed, hence the importance of opening the marrow cavity.

drilled a hole in each half. These I used to plug the cavities of the femur and tibia—the hole for the shafts of the revision prosthesis. A second head I halved and used to form new femoral condyles. Sometimes gaps needed slices of the third head.

The adult and the elderly knee

So, what are the surgical possibilities for the elderly knee? I am afraid that it very much depends upon the surgeon and his exposure to different techniques. For wear and tear osteoarthritis I favoured the hemi-arthroplasty from the beginning of the 1980s.

The majority of osteoarthritis in knees starts either under the lateral side of the patella or the medial (inside) compartment of the joint. The surgery I have just discussed.

The range of motion of hemi-arthroplasties is much better than total arthroplasties (TKRs): 120 degrees or more of flexion for a hemi compared to about 110 degrees with a total knee prosthesis. My population of elderly Italian ladies needed to be able to kneel in church and crawl around their gardens tending to the tomatoes. I saw a number of ladies who had total knee prostheses put in at 'St Elsewhere' and for whom it was too late. One can simply revise a unicompartmental to a total but not the other way around.

It sounds as though I did not do any total knee prostheses. I did a lot. The indications were really age, degree of deformation and, very importantly, the quality of the recipient bone and severity of the arthritis. Diseases like rheumatoid and gout or pseudo-gout—where there is a major disease process in the synovium, increased blood flow in the bones and osteoporosis (loss of calcium)—need total joints.

So what are the potential managements for failing adult knees with a specific arthritic process secondary to a definite disease like rheumatoid arthritis or psoriatic arthritis, where the synovium inside the joint overreacts and starts to destroy the joint surfaces?

We used to do open synovectomies and then, as arthroscopic equipment became better, arthroscopic removal of the synovium. Synovectomy and rehabilitation can buy time, particularly if good chemical or medical control of the underlying disease is achieved. This was eventually followed by joint replacement, usually a total joint. The quality of the bone is poor after years of hyperaemia (increased blood flow) in the bone triggered by the inflammatory response and the synovial disease processes, which will continue if any hyaline cartilage is left, its degeneration products being one of the triggers to the synovial reaction.

In the wear and tear osteoarthritis, which is much the most common, there is choice. One school of orthopaedics lets the knee degenerate to the point that the patient can no longer stand it, offering painkillers—which is the norm in UK practice—rather than non-steroidal anti-inflammatory medications (NSAIDs because the Americans talk about 'drugs') which was my preference. Physiotherapy does not do much to alleviate the progression of the disease.

In the 1960s, before NSAIDs were available and chemical control of the processes were poor, I recall some rheumatoid patients being obliged to take up to twenty 350mg tablets of aspirin per day to control their inflammation.

Omeprazol is a medication that seems to protect the stomach from the side-effects of oral NSAIDs: heartburn. I strongly recommend its use.

Intra-articular injections of a steroid is very helpful in some cases to gain some degree of control over the inflammatory response, always backed up with a course of NSAIDs. Physiotherapy is also needed. One could often buy a number of years this way before a more interventionalist procedure. Adding together modalities achieves a summation of effect; the whole is greater than the sum of the parts.

Arthroscopic washouts

I never offered an arthroscopy and washout of the knee, and the current literature on the subject says that they were a complete waste of time and funds! A good clinician can make a very good diagnosis from the patient's history and a careful clinical examination. Arthroscopy should be aimed at being therapeutic.

Incisions

These are not often discussed with patients, but they can have a big effect on the outcome. My wife had the temerity to ask a surgeon which approach he was proposing to use for a total hip. We had only just seen him and he was asking her to sign a consent form. When challenged to do the recommended approach, he turned on his heel and left. Was he an inadequate surgeon, old-fashioned and closed to modern thinking, or just not very manually dexterous? (Some of the world's most renowned surgeons can barely 'cut their way out of a wet paper bag with a pair of sharp scissors'. Some were reported as taking up to six hours for a primary total hip!)

It is your knee; have no qualms to ask questions like, 'How are you going to remove and reattach the quadriceps to the patella?', 'Have you considered the infrapatellar incision?' and 'I would prefer the classical Timbrel-Fisher to the midline!' Keep the surgeon on his toes!

Young surgeons, it is very much worth remembering that bone heals to bone. Muscle and tendon do not heal anything like as well. It was my practice to try to remove muscle with a shaving of bone or to use an infrapatellar incision, leaving the muscles attached to the patella. It makes the rehabilitation quicker. Muscle tissue without tendon does not hold sutures well. The repairs are therefore weaker. I would drill small holes through the bone for sutures and use slow-absorbing suture material.

The Elmslie-Trillat-Maquet realignment and elevation of the tibial tubercle can be done through a short (75 mm) curved oblique incision, most of the cutting of bone being subcutaneous. One needs to be dexterous and have sharp, thin osteotomes, and be patient cutting the bone gently from the top down and then medially on repeat passes. If you need a long midline incision, get off the pot and send the patient to someone more skilled. Ladies do not appreciate big scars on their legs from poor surgical skills.

Notes for the Health Care Practitioner's Attention and to Raise the Patient's Expectations as to What Might be Reasonably Expected

Examination of the knee

This I admit is aimed at the practising professional and not at the suffering lay reader, but I believe that this is what you can expect.

> *'Art is the perception and manipulation of parameters that*
> *science cannot measure.'*
> (I attribute this to myself.)

Better clinical examination skills of patients might yield a more subtle understanding of the knee.

The jingo learned at medical school was, 'Inspection, palpation, percussion and auscultation; these are the basis of a good examination', and while having a nice rhythmic ring to them when chanted, it does not quite work for the knees. Look, feel, move, active movements and passive, please, are rather more appropriate.

Examination of the knee requires one to see not just the knees but also the quadriceps of the thighs; so, patient, you do need to be able to take off trousers, or wear a skirt. It was extraordinary how often people were unprepared for this. Most professionals will have developed their own rituals, but this is what one can expect, and challenge anything less.

I would immediately feel for the flexibility of the metacarpal joints and pinch up the skin on the dorsum of the hand; it gave me an impression of the individual's flexibility or natural laxity that might be in their joints.

Look at the alignment of the legs, not only lying on the examination couch but also standing. Quite often as a patient moves from one position to another—climbing onto or off the examination couch or putting a leg into a trouser—one can see abnormal movements like anterior/posterior displacement of the femoral condyle on the tibial plateau, even if later examination for these abnormalities is difficult because the patient cannot fully relax.

A common sight is an apparently 'straight' leg on the examination table becoming a bit more bow-legged when standing. (Note that this also occurs in X-ray machines.) The medial compartment damage starts to show up, Wolff's law. Look for any scarring.

Look at the bulk of the quadriceps, and in particular look at the bulk of the vastus medialis oblique on both the good side and the painful side. And then look for QIS, delay of the VMO when contracting the quadricep muscle group.

I suggest gentle palpation of any area that is indicated as painful. Localisation of the patient's site of pain is most important. Think of the underlying structures. Is the joint swollen and warm or is it cool? Are the tissues boggy or normal? Unfortunately, many knees are rather well padded, which can make for difficulty.

Palpate for fluid. A dry joint means that the hyaline cartilage is 'happy'; fluid in the joint means that the surfaces somewhere are less than 'happy'. This does not always correspond to the patient's presentation! Persistent fluid in a joint is often the indication for an arthroscopy in combination with other clinical findings.

Sometimes it is better to ask the patient to make active movements prior to further passive tests if the patient seems a bit timorous. In particular, ask the patient to contract their quadriceps with the leg straight lying of the examination couch. One can often see a slight delay in the activity of the VMO: QIS.

Well, sometimes. If you note there is slight delay in the VMO with reference to the other muscles, this is possibly the most important and least often looked for sign of slight quadricep incoordination. Rectifying this slight delay is the cure for so many knee problems: VMO instruction and review in two to three weeks.

Movements

Initially, do these with one's hands on the joint, feeling for crepitations, grindings, 'snaps', 'crackles' or 'pops'. One puts the knee through as full a range of motion as possible, passively and then actively.

And then the 'specialist' tests:

- With the knee straight, or almost straight, test for the integrity of the medial and lateral collateral ligaments.
- The McMurray manoeuvre was what we used to call bending to full rollback position, twisting the fully flexed knee by twisting the foot in and out and then partially straightening it, to try to pick up the torn meniscus. It is a knack, but it is a jolly useful test. One can determine medial or lateral meniscal damage.

Tests for cruciate ligament instability

There are various tests for cruciate ligament damage. (The 'pros' know all about them, 'cause there's money to be made.)

For the posterior cruciate, just bend the knee to 90 degrees and gently push backwards with the examiner's thumbs on the joint line. In a normal knee the tibial plateau is always a little forward of the femoral condyle; the knee is after all towards the rollback position. If the PCL (posterior cruciate ligament) is torn, the tibial plateau edge is below or behind the femoral condyles. It is as simple as that.

For the ACL there are various ways of trying to demonstrate if the tibial plateau and femoral condyle fall out of alignment in the relaxed straight leg. The femoral condyle falls backwards from over the tibial plateau with the knee extended. As the knee is bent, the plateau jumps back under the femoral condyles. Patients find this distressing and often become too tense to be examined. This so-called Pivot Shift[23] test or 'jerk sign or test' was only described in the late 1960s. Before that the diagnosis of a cruciate ligament damage was not made.

After some years as a consultant I was shown a test for the ACL done with the ankle under the examiner's arm: foot in the armpit, the leg over the examiner's forearm, the opposite hand on the lateral side of the leg just below the knee and the hand from under the leg holding the examiner's wrist. It is a sort of figure-of-four position.

For the left knee, face the patient and put the left foot and ankle under the left arm with one's forearm under the patient's calf. Place one's right hand over the head of the fibula and grasp one's right wrist with the left hand.

One has very firm control of the leg and can move the knee very gently—no jerks or uncomfortable moments. It is by far the best test for ACL instability.

After that, one should look at radiographs: AP and lateral views, but also an AP view weight-bearing, to show if the medial compartment closes, implying that the hyaline cartilage is worn away and looking to see if the bone is denser in the medial tibial plateau—Wolff's sign. It implies that the bone is working harder (i.e. taking more load).

A skyline patellar view looks at the shape of that bone and the state of the medial and lateral articular facet of the bone. If there is wear, hooking of osteophytes and increased density of the bone on the lateral side, one is looking at osteoarthritic development. Alignment is rather a dynamic thing, and really one cannot lay too much store by these views for alignment.

---

[23] In the knee with intact cruciate ligaments, they act as the pivot when the tibia and femur rotate in respect to each other in their long axis. When there is a cruciate ligament rupture, the axis of rotation immediately becomes the medial collateral ligament. The axis, or pivot, has shifted.

Good rehabilitation of the VMO can change things in functional mode, even for the early mildly arthritic patellofemoral joint.

Occasionally, there is a place for a 'through notch' view and even oblique views. These can show osteophytosis on the notch blocking extension and can help confirming the suspicion of a loose body hiding in a corner.

As a result of my years in Canada, I would also do the routine rheumatology blood tests and joint aspiration if I thought it necessary. After all, for the patient 'one-stop shopping' is more convenient, and the system only paid out one consultation fee; follow-up fees were very meagre. I

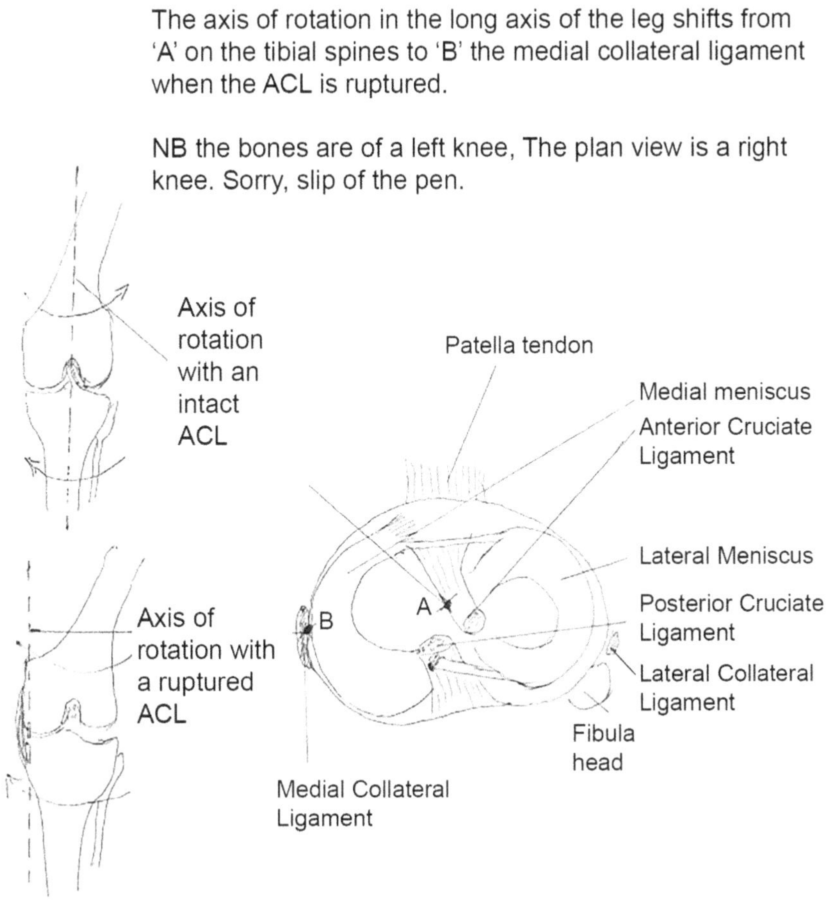

The axis of rotation in the long axis of the leg shifts from 'A' on the tibial spines to 'B' the medial collateral ligament when the ACL is ruptured.

NB the bones are of a left knee, The plan view is a right knee. Sorry, slip of the pen.

Axis of rotation with an intact ACL

Patella tendon

Medial meniscus
Anterior Cruciate Ligament

Lateral Meniscus

Axis of rotation with a ruptured ACL

B   A

Posterior Cruciate Ligament

Lateral Collateral Ligament

Fibula head

Medial Collateral Ligament

Fig 52 Pivot shift

would try, and I would instruct my trainees, to add as much value at each visit as possible. Clinics can get blocked up so easily without these disciplines. (In my northern UK area, the iatrogenic effect of still being "under the hospital" was not to be underestimated!)

SCANS! 'I need a scan ...'

MRI scans are expensive, flattering, popular and confusing: false positives and false negatives. One cannot see articular cartilage lesions nor synovial lesions, unless they are quite big, on any scan, and the actual edge (cortex) of the bones is not accurately displayed, as it does not have much water in it, and that is really what MRIs are looking at: water molecules. Alas, our legal friends have made them almost imperative; increased confusion and anxiety have a positive effect on legal billings.

If you can localise a site of pain, think about what structures might be there. An effusion in a joint means that some part of the surface is not happy and the synovium is having to work overtime. For me, an effusion is the indication for an arthroscopy in someone who could otherwise be expected to have a normal knee. On the other hand, an elderly person with obvious arthritis on clinical examination and X-ray films is not going to be helped at all by a washout arthroscopy; recent published papers have shown this to be a complete waste of time and money. Their problem needs correct medication and probably some form of surgery, such as a replacement arthroplasty.

Clinicians need to examine their patients, not just test them! Tests do not treat!

Tissue and flexibility

People are built very differently, not only in their shapes but also in the flexibility of their tissues. When examining an orthopaedic patient, I make a point of noting just how flexible their tissues are by gently pinching and lifting the skin on the dorsum (back) of the hand and bending their fingers backwards gently. With time, one gets a feel for the differences. Does this hyper-flexibility matter? Yes and no.

Collagen is the fibrous protein that holds the body together. There are different forms of collagen and some of them are more stretchy than others. People with the condition of Ehlers-Danlos syndrome have very poor-quality collagen, which results in laxity of tissues, tendons, joints and other collagen structures. Their problems and control probably lie outside the scope of this book.

Those people with ligaments on the lax side of normal with very flexible joints can function perfectly normally. This is because most of our movement patterns are brought about by coordinated muscle movements and do not rely on ligaments. (I have gone so far as to state that in my view the anterior cruciate and the posterior cruciate ligaments are there not to control movement but to ensure that the bones, tibia and femur, are aligned correctly at the moment of initiating a movement. They hold the bones aligned while we are asleep or relaxed. They occasionally avulse or tear under load, and hence the very profitable industry in their repair.)

Very stretchy ligaments can make a difference to the technical aspects of reconstruction for ligament instability. But the principles of rehabilitation, of improving muscle coordination post-op, are the same in all cases.

Some problems of repair and healing tend to be the production of tough, inflexible scar tissue, which is collagen fibres but laid down in a haphazard fashion. The natural history of scar tissue is to shrink with time; to shrink to the point that the small capillaries and blood vessels in the scar tissue become choked off, resulting in hard, ischaemic, contracted tissue and occasionally even ectopic calcification. Excision of this sort of scar tissue is sometimes indicated if it is causing painful contracture. On the other hand, the contraction can be used to the advantage of the repair.

> The classic Girdlestone salvage procedure for a failed hip was simply excision of the remains of the joint and permitting nature to form scar tissue. One had to hold the limb in the right orientation vis-à-vie rotation. The results of Girdlestone salvage procedures were much better after an infection. Infection is a big stimulus to inflammation and scarring. The result can be a solid hip, shortened but strong enough to walk on.
>
> A similar procedure can be used in the shoulder to very good effect. I had a patient who worked as a volunteer in the hospital shop. She had a failed shoulder prosthesis removed, which I left as an excision arthroplasty because of infection. She was very happy to be demonstrated to the trainee surgeons, most of whom missed the fact that she did not have a shoulder joint at all until they saw the X-rays. She had a surprisingly full range of motion, including being able to do her hair, and apparently normal power.

Excision arthroplasty is not an option in the knee, as it is essentially one bone—the femur— sitting on top of the other—the tibia. There is no boney socket. The 'socket' is the hood of the anteromedial and anterolateral capsule, the retinacula and the collateral ligaments, the patella and the patellar tendon and the vastus medialis oblique muscle, which controls the tension in those structures.

So, are flexible ligaments a problem or not? Yes, the examining clinician can overdiagnose instability if he does not examine both sides; but no, not really from the surgical point of view. More important to recovery is good rehabilitation, strengthening and coordinating the controlling muscles post any sort of repair.

Continuous passive motion (CPM) and movement

Continuous passive motion is applied as a therapeutic concept to limb injury and in particular to joint injury. In the early 1970s one Dr Robert Salter, working in Toronto, Canada, injected staphylococcus into healthy rabbit knees. Some he moved immediately, some he moved after a delay of a three or four days and some he did not move at all for three weeks.

He found that in those knees that did not move, there was complete lysis (melting away) of the hyaline articular joint surfaces: that is, a complete destruction of the joint surface by the toxins and enzymes released by the bacteria.

In those rabbit knees where there was a three-day delay before movement, there was some lysis of the hyaline articular cartilage but there was then a development of fibrocartilage as a form of repair.

In those that were moved immediately from the time of the injection of the bacteria, he claimed that there was preservation of the hyaline articular cartilage.

Unfortunately, I believe, for the UK population, when he was invited to present his results in this country, he was felt to be a bit lightweight and possibly economical with the truth. In short, the establishment of orthopaedic consultants had him down as a 'bullshitter' and CPM did not get the attention it deserves.

The understanding of the physiology of cartilage and the physical conditions necessary for its maintenance in good health was completely ignored by most practising orthopaedic consultants during my professional life from 1968 to 2006. Even to this day, many proposed solutions to osteoarthritis and cartilage loss fly in the face of what is known. (Cartilage physiology is discussed in Section 2.)

Of equal importance, but not confined to UK orthopaedics, is the idea that hyaline cartilage cannot heal. It is a demonstration of 'derivative thinking'. This seems to have arisen in the 1950s and 1960s and has been promulgated from orthopaedic text to orthopaedic text unquestioned. I have discussed it elsewhere. In fact, cartilage cells have a very slow metabolism, and very rarely do they need to divide, but they can if necessary, during growth for example.

I believe that under the right physical conditions of pressure, movement, lack of shear and perhaps patient nutrition articular cartilage can heal with something very like hyaline cartilage. The point is that if the right physical conditions are restored, hyaline articular cartilage has an ability to heal. This is what Dr Salter demonstrated with CPM, which is one of the reasons I believe CPM is so valuable.

CPM is also beneficial at a number of levels in limb rehabilitation:

a) Less analgesia. It was noted that patients on CPM require much less analgesia post-operatively, and often none at all. There are none of the risks of overmedication: immobility, poor respiratory excursion and pressure sores from lying immobile. They are not drugged to mask the discomfort that prevents the patient from moving.

b) Soft tissue healing. Not only do the articular surfaces benefit from movement, the other soft tissues—skin, capsule, tendons, muscles—seem to benefit and heal better.

c) Bone healing is improved.

d) There is less muscle atrophy.

e) Less requirement for physiotherapy time.

f) There is, on theoretical grounds, less risk of deep venous thrombosis.

g) Increase of patient stimulation. In this world of limited resources, the act of moving the CPM machine from patient to patient ensures two or four more visits and stimulation of the patient by staff per day.

In my practice, I used it in treating the elderly patient after a hip operation, even for a fracture, to gain these hidden benefits. We also used a Do-It-Yourself system for hip and knee surgery when all orthopaedic beds had Balkan beams over them as a routine. It was a simple matter to rig up a Thomas splint with a Pearson knee piece under the leg and give the patients the pieces of cord to pull. The more these patients could take some responsibility for their rehabilitation, the better they seemed to do. And it required less staff time. The Balkan beam carried a 'monkey bar', which also permitted the patient to use their arms to move in the bed. Usually, there was a degree of elevation of the foot of the bed, which makes sitting up in bed easier and speeds the venous return, and as Virchow pointed out, this is one of the most important things necessary to reduce the risk of blood clotting in the leg veins: the dreaded and dangerous deep venous thrombosis.

I used CPM quite often when I did a patelloplasty: that is, turning the patella over and cutting off the osteophytes and even the eburnated bone to expose the cancellous bone of the interior of the patella. This was on the lateral facet. Following a few days of CPM these patients go on to recover what appears to be normal patellofemoral function. Whether they formed new hyaline cartilage surfaces or fibrocartilage surfaces I do not know.

CPM is also available for upper limb use. Although I recall using it, I cannot recall details. It is a useful adjunct to post-op healing. About 45 seconds of cycling time and about 30 degree of range to start with increasing toward 90 degrees of motion. We had a limited number of machines, so they were moved around: two-hour sessions for each patient, but loads of patient stimulation.

Some Surgical Procedures and Reflections Thereon

———•———

For those who need to know, read on, but for the lay minded, skip all this.

Fractured patella

The treatment for this is dependent upon just how much damage is produced, in particular how much damage to the weight-bearing articular surfaces and the degree of displacement of the bits. Steps in articular surfaces following fractures in any joint are to be avoided, as they lead to osteoarthritic changes with joint surface destruction, sometimes quite quickly. It is the role of the bonesetter today to reduce the fragments as far as is possible.

Obviously, if there is just a crack (technical term 'fissure') visible on the radiographs, little needs to be done. The fragments will be held together by the soft tissue envelope. It is when there is tearing of the soft tissue envelope, such that the bone fragments can displace one from the other, that some form of surgical reduction becomes necessary. This is true of all fractures.

Tension band wire

The surgical treatment advised for multiple fragments is tension band wiring, where the fracture site can be pulled apart by muscle contraction. Occasionally some fragments are so small that they need to be removed.

In the case of the knee, after wound cleaning and debridement, and these are often open injuries from road traffic accidents, the pieces of patella are manipulated back into position and held with a couple of bone clamps. Two parallel pins are passed through the pieces (this needs a drill normally) in the same alignment as the long axis of the leg. A fairly thin stainless-steel wire is then wound around the pin ends in a figure of eight. This permits the forces to bypass the fracture site and also holds the fragments against the femoral surfaces.

It is essential to start very early movement, even if it is only a jog initially. To this end a light Jones bandage and a CPM machine are ideal. The early movement seems to stimulate the chondrocytes to make an effort. Many hold that hyaline cartilage cannot heal, but good quality fibrocartilage can substitute (see discussion in Section 2 'What is meant by Movement?').

Once healed, the wire and the pins are removed.

Patellectomy

When there is massive destruction of the patella, a very dirty wound and loss of pieces, patellectomy used to be recommended. This entailed the complete removal of the fragments of the patella and a sort of cobbled, crossover of the remains of the tendon ends. Traditionally, this was held straight for four to six weeks in a cylinder cast or a Robert Jones bandage. Interestingly, these tendons did heal, and with time they actually thickened and strengthened to be fully functional. The final thickness of the patella/quadricep tendon will be about the same as the thickness of the patella. Just how long this hypertrophy and thickening takes is difficult to say, but probably the best part of three years from injury and repair.

I have seen a number of patients subjected to this treatment, some with virtually normal function but more with problems (perhaps because the functional ones did not need to see an orthopaedic surgeon?). Their problems ranged from weakness—of the leg 'giving way' and rather non-specific anterior knee pain on walking or on stairs—to neuroma-like pain causing major disability.

Thinking neuroma, trying to identify the site and then removal of the neuroma is paramount. At the same time, a little bit of synovitis from low-grade osteoarthritis can be a source of pain from trapping of the synovial fimbriae (it looks a bit like seaweed with the arthroscope) that can develop. Simple removal is needed, followed by quadricep rehabilitation.

For a number of patients just VMO rehabilitation was enough; they could reawaken their VMO muscle when shown how. Of interest is that the muscle is still there, and it can be reawakened to function normally after years of underuse, although it may take a little time.

Patelloplasty

This is probably a point of controversy with many surgeons unfamiliar with the technique, but it is a very valid and useful operation whereby the osteophytes and damaged articular surfaces of the patella are debrided and the shape may have to be altered to permit the bone to align in the intercondylar notch. This is particularly necessary with a realignment procedure like the Elmslie-Trillat-Maquet. I have described them above.

Surgical approaches to the knee

The knee is quite a sensitive place to have an operation; one of the advantages of arthroscopic surgery is that the wounds are so much smaller and the pain much less.

Looking at the knee from the front, the medial side seems much more sensitive than the lateral side. This is presuming the surgeon has the skill and whit to avoid the infrapatellar nerve.

The surgical approach for these sorts of procedures is the medial parapatellar incision described by Timbrel-Fisher. More recently a midline straight incision of the skin is used by many. Both leave ugly scars. See Langer's lines below.

The detachment of the vastus medialis oblique from the patella, and more importantly its reattachment on closure of the wound, is, I think, poorly performed by many surgeons. Some surgeons just cut it off and cobble it back expecting it to heal!

Bone heals to bone well; some advocate cutting off flakes of bone with the muscle's fibrous insertion, some cut within the fibrous insertion and some, I am sad to say, just cut the muscle. Muscle almost never heals to bone, and muscle is very poorly held by sutures. This really is poor surgical technique (offered, I might add, in 2012 to a member of my family). My preference was to take flakes of bone and drill small holes in the patella to reattach.

Infrapatellar approach

Some operative dissections can be done without detaching the VMO, but they do need a lot of freeing up of the muscle and retraction of the muscle, which can cause it damage. Bleeding can occur from the anastomosing arteries on the medial side and can cause a disastrous haematoma post-op!

Post-op in my view is to encourage immediate movement with quadriceps and VMO training. Some patients need CPM, but most can go home almost immediately.

There are now more, clever surgeons and smaller incisions.

Reasons why the hemi-Marmor was so good

The main proviso is that the surgeon had to be good enough to 'eyeball' what he was doing. There were no real jigs in the modern sense. Jigs rely on there being a cortex that has been evolved to weight-bear.

The placement of the femoral portion was critical to include not only the size but the direction on the bone, angled to follow the orientation of the condyle. A narrow V-shaped trough was cut and a hole drilled for the 'keel'. This should be almost a perfect press fit, although a small amount of cement was used.

The top of the tibia was prepared by removing the upper surface of the tibial plateau but retaining a rim of cortex and a little cancellous bone. A fine burr was very useful, as were fine SHARP osteotomes. Again, a press fit was best. And then the two bits were cemented in.

It worked because of the following:

- No restraints on sliding forwards, backwards or in rotation.
- The company, Richards, used a pressure technique for making the tibial plateau block and a sterilisation technique that resulted in a high-density polyethylene relatively resistant to shear and flaking. Other companies' products were discovered to flake and break up.
- The tibial plateau was let into and supported on the cancellous bone of the plateau. The load was transferred as nature intended by the hydraulic effect of incompressible fat and blood. There could be a visible line of 'loosening' under the tibial component in a perfectly functioning knee.

Other products were developed to be sat on the cortical rim, partly to permit jigs to be used in achieving alignment. The cortex of the tibial plateau was not evolved to be weight-bearing but to resist bursting, to contain the hydraulic pressure from within.

(In choosing your surgeon, ask if he needs to use jigs. He will not like it but it is a reflection of just what sort of technical hands he has! A good few 'jigged' attempts have I had to diddle with to get right when called in to help others.)

I recall a meeting, late 1979, where the injection of cement into the cancellous bone was being advocated as improving the fixation of the tibial side of a knee replacement. However, on opening the discussion of the advisability of the technique, the moderator, Dr Jo Miller, an advocate and a major researcher in the field, actually stopped and gave serious consideration to the suggestion that it might not be the ideal way to transfer the load into the proximal tibia.

Langer's lines

These describe the alignment of the collagen fibres in the skin. It used to be taught that surgical incisions must be parallel to Langer's line. Certainly, if they are, the wounds tend to be thinner with less keloid.

Modern surgeons often use midline incisions over the knee, something I avoided. It is something one might discuss with one's surgeon.

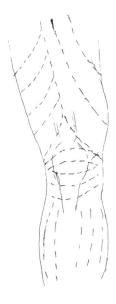

Langer's Lines

Around the front of the knee, sometimes known as cleavage lines, they are to do with the general alignment of the collagen fibres in the dermis.

Incisions that follow Langer's Lines tend to make for better scars.

Fig 53 Langer's lines

Glossary of Terms

Albumin: a protein in blood with a large molecular weight of about 64,000 g/mol.

Anecdote: Anecdotes are anathema to the academic medical world which has become fixated on the reporting of results and 'met-analysis', meaning the pooling of ever larger numbers of reported results from different papers. To stand up at a meeting and try to pass comment exampling one or two cases that do not seem to fit the reported pattern will just bring derision from the less experienced. The scientific method starts with observation, from which one hypothesises. This is followed by experimentation, to prove or disprove, and then theorisation.

Anterior Superior Iliac Spine (ASIS): a bony landmark at the front of the iliac crest of the pelvis.

Arthroscope: a narrow-bored tube with lenses for looking into joints, usually with a camera attached and the view displayed on a TV screen. Specially designed instruments for working in the confined space of a joint have been developed. Arthroscopy is the surgical procedure of using an arthroscope.

Arthrotomy: an incision into a joint.

Arthroplasty: the operation of implanting an artificial joint prosthesis into a joint.

Articularis genu: a small muscle deep under the front group of the thigh that pulls the knee joint capsule up so that it does not get trapped as the knee goes from flexed to straight.

Axon: the main connection fibre of a nerve cell. Some are long and some are short, depending on their situation.

Baker's cyst: a synovial-lined swelling behind the knee that can develop in an arthritic knee.

Biofeedback: in this context, the act of having the finger on the muscle tells the brain what is actually happening and not what it thinks is happening.

Carrying angle: the fixed angle of the thigh bone with the leg bone.

Chondrocalcinosis: ectopic calcification in tissue. Ectopic means 'outside its normal place'. Multiple causes.

Chondrocyte: a cartilage cell.

Chondrosarcoma: a rare cancer of cartilage cells.

Collateral ligaments: ligaments at the side of a joint—in the knee, medial and lateral—responsible for stability.

Compliance: medical use means that patients go on doing what they have been told to do!

Condyle, femoral: medial and lateral, the articular facets of the distal femur.

Concentric: contraction (shortening) of muscle under load.

Continuous Passive Movement (CPM): there are machines that move the limb slowly and continuously after a surgical procedure. Things heal quicker and pain is reduced. Very beneficial.

Deep Venous Thrombosis (DVT): clotting in the deep veins of the calf and leg. It can be painful and can also be very dangerous. If a blood clot that is not attached to the vein wall breaks off, it is swept to the heart's right side, where it is then swept through and can block off the pulmonary artery. It can cause a reflex nervous effect that can stop the heart. Death from a pulmonary embolus is the expected outcome.

Dendrite: connection fibres of nerve cells, secondary to the main axon.

Diarthrodial joint: all the joints in the body that move. Always two hyaline surfaces opposed to each other.

Diffusion: the passive mechanism whereby molecules distribute themselves through a solution. Usually, it is from a high concentration to a lower concentration.

Eccentric: extension and elongation of a muscle under load.

Electromyelogram (EMG): a diagnostic procedure to assess the health of muscles and the nerve cells that control them (motor neurons). EMG results can reveal nerve dysfunction, muscle dysfunction or problems with nerve-to-muscle signal transmission.

Elmslie-Trillat-Maquet: a combination of a surgical realignment and elevation of the tibial tubercle for patellofemoral problems.

Equinus: the position of the foot pointing downwards, from the manner in which a horse walks on its toenails.

Facet: an articular surface covered with hyaline cartilage.

Fascia lata (and tensor fascia latae): a tough, thick fascial band and its muscle that stabilises the quads on the lateral (outside) of the thigh.

Fibrinogen: a circulating protein that is the precursor of fibrin that forms blood clots. It can be labelled with iodine (I_{131}) and was used extensively in medical research years ago.

Fibroblast: a cell that turns into a fibrocyte that can produce collagen fibres. In healing, they line up and are said to 'palisade'.

Fibrocartilage: a surface material produced by chondrocytes as a form of healing after a period of delay in movement of an articular surface. There is more fibrous material in it and it wears poorly by comparison with hyaline cartilage.

Foreign body: medical term for anything foreign in the body, deliberate or accidental.

Gerdy's tubercle: attachment of the fascia lata, front lateral side of the upper tibia.

Glycosaminoglycans (GAGs): chondroitin sulphate in children and keratin sulphate in adults. Constituent chemicals in the matrix of hyaline cartilage.

Gracilis: a muscle on the inside of the thigh. Part of the hamstrings.

Hamstrings: the muscles at the back of the thigh that bend the knee and help control rotation of the femur on the tibia.

Hemi-Marmor prosthesis: the first unicompartmental knee prosthesis.

Hunter's cap: a malformation of the patella that develops without significant vastus medialis oblique pull.

Hyaline cartilage: the shiny, smooth, articular surface material in all joints. Visible in any butcher's shop.

Hyaluronic acid: an important constituent molecule of synovial fluid and cartilage. It is a good lubricant.

Iatrogenic: induced by the medical process. *Iatros* = doctor in Greek.

Inflammatory response: the manner in which the body's tissues respond to any trauma: radiation, physical, chemical, heat. The capillaries start to leak fluid from the blood into the tissues between the cells. It is the cause of swelling and is obligatory in the first five or six days. It can be reduced by generous use of ice.

Isometric: muscle contraction but with no movement.

Isotonic: muscle working with the same load through a range of movement.

Langer's lines: the orientation of the collagen fibres in skin.

Linea aspera: a ridge down the back of the femur to which muscles attach.

Lumen: medical word for the hole down the centre of any blood vessel.

Lymphocyte: a white cell that concerns itself with immunity.

Matrix: the substance of the cartilage, chondrocytes and collagen fibres in a solution of hyaluronic acid with chondroitin or keratin sulphate attached; essentially, joint fluid or synovial fluid.

McMurray sign: a manoeuvre of the knee to indicate a torn meniscus.

Meniscus: fibrocartilaginous C-shaped entities in the knee that fill the space between the curved femoral condyles and the flatter tibial surfaces.

Milieu intérieur: Claude Bernard's concept of the local environment of a cell at the cellular level.

Motor unit: the number of muscle fibres supplied by a single nerve axon.

Neutrophil: a white cell that has amoeba-like ability to ingest and destroy dead tissue and foreign tissue like bacteria.

NSAIDs: non-steroidal anti-inflammatory drugs.

Oblique line: a ridge on the front of the upper femur, origin of the vastus medialis and intermedius muscles.

Omeprazole: a medication that protects the stomach from irritation by acid and NSAIDs.

Osmosis: the physical phenomenon of solute molecules passing from a low concentration into a higher concentration when the solutions are separated by a semi-permeable membrane that does not permit the passage of the dissolved molecules. It is the number of molecules, not the size of the dissolved molecules, that is important.

Osteocyte: a bone cell.

Osteomyelitis: infection in the bone, quite common prior to the era of antibiotics. Treatment was surgical incision and drainage with months of healing by secondary intention.

Osteophytes: bony projections from the weight-bearing areas that are covered in hyaline cartilage that seem to be an attempt at repair in osteoarthritic joints.

Pathology: the medical term for something being wrong with a part of the body.

Patelloplasty: an operation to modify the shape of the undersurface of the patella.

Patterning: the position assumed by the decerebrate body, when the brain's motor cortex is no longer connected to the spinal cord. It is the result of the spinal reflexes, flexion of the arms and full extension of the legs.

Phase: in this sense, flexion phase or extension phase.

Physiology: the chemistry of the working of the body.

Plateau: upper tibial articular facets, medial and lateral.

Poliomyelitis: a viral disease that is endemic in the Middle East, meaning that it was common. It kills the motor-neurone cells in the spinal cord, resulting in paralysis.

Proteoglycans (PG): Hyaluronic acid in synovial fluid.

Prosthesis: a mechanical device, such as a total joint.

Prosthetic: something removeable like a knee brace or a wrist splint.

'Q' Angle: the angle in the pulley system of the quads and the patella and patellar tendon, which is constantly changing.

Quadricep Incoordination Syndrome (QIS): the clinical finding of a delay in contraction of the VMO in relation to contraction of the other quadricep muscle—not yet described in medical literature.

Quadriceps: the muscles of the front of the thigh that are essentially involved in straightening the knee.

Rectus femoris: classified as a quadricep but also crosses the hip joint.

Retinaculum: thickened bands of the knee joint capsule that act like ligaments; medial and lateral.

Secondary intention: wound healing where the wound is left open and the skin is prevented from growing over the pathological tissue that has been surgically exposed and excised. The body produces granulation tissue, which gradually fills the wound, and eventually the skin is permitted to grow over it. A slow process.

Sartorius: muscle in front of the thigh, probably a stabiliser of the quads' mass.

Skyline view: special X-ray view of the patella (see diagram on page 92).

Soleus: one of the calf muscles. It does not cross the knee. Gastrocnemius does cross the knee.

Spina bifida: failure of the spinal canal to form normally during foetal growth, resulting in degrees of paralysis below the affected level.

Subtalar joint: the joint in the hindfoot under the talus. At the front, the head of the talus articulates with the cuneiform medially and at the back of the body it articulates with the calcaneus. This permits our feet to twist to accommodate uneven ground, but the axis of the joint is about 13 degrees upwards and outwards so the foot is twisted as the joint moves and this causes the tibia to rotate.

Synovium: the membrane lining a joint. Some cells secrete synovial fluid and some are responsible for clearing up any debris.

Synovectomy: operation of removing the synovium from a joint.

TENS machine: transcutaneous electrical nerve stimulation. A device to control pain. The mechanism of function is not entirely clear. It seems to be entirely safe. Turned up high it can trigger muscle twitching.

Tibial tubercle or tibial tuberosity: attachment of the patellar tendon onto the tibia.

Tibialis posterior: a powerful extensor and inverter of the foot whose tendon is deep behind the ankle on the medial side. It tends to get forgotten.

Thomas heel: a prosthetic medial wedge for the heel of a shoe.

UHMWPE: ultra-high-density molecular-weight polyethylene. The plastic-bearing surface material. Preceded by HDMWP.

Valgus: angles laterally.

Varus: angles medially.

Vastus intermedius: a major straightener of the knee.

Vastus lateralis: the biggest of the power muscles straightening the knee.

Vastus medialis: a straightener of the knee.

Vastus medialis oblique (VMO): part of the quadriceps, but with steering function, not power. Hero of this book.

Venous thrombosis: clotting of blood in a vein (see DVT).

Virchow's triad: the postulate that three conditions contributed to DVT: 1. changes in the chemistry of the blood, intrinsic; 2. damage to the blood vessel wall, extrinsic; or 3. stasis, reduced or absent blood flow.

Wolff's sign: a radiological sign of increased bone density in the loaded area. In the knee it is usually the medial tibial plateau. It suggests that the bone is working hard.

Author Biography

Mr Hedley Piper, FRCS is a retired UK consultant orthopaedic surgeon. He trained in the NHS of the early 1970s. It was a surprisingly wide general surgical exposure. At 30 with his fellowship, he moved to practise for four years as a surgeon GP in a remote town in central British Columbia, Canada. (There was a rock at the roadside testifying to this.) Fielding all the trauma of logging, farming, mining and many miles of open, unpaved roads proved the benefit of those long hours at the NHS coal face. 'Trauma' took on new perspectives! Obstetrics and gynaecology, autopsy and social pathology were all in a day's work.

He refocused on orthopaedic surgery in 1978; three years of residency at McGill, Montreal, required a greater focus on the obscure details of orthopaedic pathologies. There was a lot to read and ingest. Then married with two children and nearly 10 years of very general orthopaedic practice in Montreal, hovering on the edge of academia but having to make a living, he returned to the UK in 1992 and was appointed as a consultant orthopaedic surgeon in Yorkshire.

The irony of orthopaedic surgery is that it is the management of multiple aches and pains not really covered in formal orthopaedic training, possibly because those teaching and writing the books were still too young to actually have experienced aches and pains. The ideas in this book are based on 35 years of continuous and varied surgical practice—the problems of the knee being but a small part.

Milton Keynes UK
Ingram Content Group UK Ltd.
UKHW020213141023
430515UK00002B/3